Thromboembolism in Orthopedic Surgery

Juan V. Llau

Editor

Thromboembolism in Orthopedic Surgery

Springer

Editor
Juan V. Llau, M.D., Ph.D.
Department of Anaesthesiology
and Critical Care
University Hospital of Valencia
Valencia
Spain

ISBN 978-1-4471-4335-2   ISBN 978-1-4471-4336-9   (eBook)
DOI 10.1007/978-1-4471-4336-9
Springer London Heidelberg New York Dordrecht

Library of Congress Control Number: 2012950006

Printed on acid-free paper

Springer is part of Springer Science+Business Media (www.springer.com)

Preface

Venous thromboembolism in any of its kinds of presentation, pulmonary embolism and deep vein thrombosis, represents a major public health problem, affecting hundreds of thousands of people each year. Patients undergoing major orthopedic surgery have a particularly high risk for developing venous thromboembolism, and the need for thromboprophylaxis, most commonly pharmacological prophylaxis, has become standard of care for many years.

In this field, the rationale for thromboprophylaxis has been widely demonstrated, as seen in the decrease of venographic and symptomatic deep vein thrombosis and symptomatic, asymptomatic, and fatal pulmonary embolism. But, due to the natural history of venous thromboembolism in patients undergoing major orthopedic surgery (mainly joint arthroplasty or hip fracture surgery), venous thromboembolism is still one of the most common causes for readmission to the hospital after surgery. Furthermore, venous thromboembolism continues to be reported in too much patients within the 2–3 months after the patient discharge, being most of them symptomatic.

From these preliminary statements, the question could be why venous thromboembolism is so prevalent between patients on orthopedic surgery although everybody knows that its prevention is one of the cornerstones of the care of these patients. The answer is multiple, including the difficulty to include the prevention protocols into the routine process of care, the need for improving the effectiveness of some protocols or drugs and the controversies in other ones, the historical lack of collaboration between all clinicians involved in the care of patients, the fear to the related bleeding of the administration of more effective drugs and protocols, and the doubts for thromboprophylaxis in some low- or moderate-risk procedures.

There are several guidelines available for the use of thromboprophylaxis in orthopedics published as international consensus by scientific societies (as the American College of Chest Physicians, ACCP, which updates its recommendations every 4 years) or under the support of some government (such as the National Institute of Clinical Excellence (NICE) and the Scottish Intercollegiate Guidelines Network (SIGN)) or by teams of expert authors in peer-reviewed prestigious journals. Existing guidelines should be often updated because new evidence emerges, new drugs demand a place in the protocols (as new oral anticoagulants), new effective protocols demonstrate their ability for the incorporation in the existing rules (as the extension of prophylaxis in hip arthroplasty), or the consensus moves to change the interpretation of previous studies. In certain sense, guidelines need to be updated to remain alive.

Is it necessary to review in a book all these questions to improve the application of thromboprophylaxis with the final objective to be better in this field? Probably, the book you have in your hands has been born with this high objective, with a panel of expert authors from some different medical specialities which gives to the chapters a multidisciplinary approach.

The book reviews the main topics in thromboprophylaxis around orthopedic surgery, from a general scope of the problems with the disease highlighting them in orthopedics to the new specific protocols involving, for example, new oral anticoagulants. The prevalence of the venous thromboembolism in each procedure (from "easy" to "hard" surgeries, with different rates of related thrombosis) and the risk factors to bear in mind in each one (related and nonrelated with the orthopedic procedure) are also revised. A chapter focuses on the diagnosis and treatment of venous thromboembolism, which is commonly "forgotten" in many books addressed to orthopedic surgeons and anesthesiologists. The methods for thromboprophylaxis have three specific chapters: the most common drugs used and recommended when pharmacological prophylaxis is needed, new drugs which are arising day by day and which management will be of main importance in a close near future, and mechanical methods, recommended both as additional when possible and for sole indications when the risk of bleeding could move us to minimize the real risk of thrombosis. Anesthetic implications for thromboprophylaxis and, also, main implications of the application of antithrombotic protocols in the anesthetic practice are covered by another chapter. In our opinion, it was very important to divide the orthopedic procedures according to their own thrombotic risk, so having their own protocols for thromboprophylaxis, high-risk, day surgery procedures, and "special" surgical procedures are included in three different chapters, from three different authors with complementary views. Finally, in the last chapter, we review the problems involving the perioperatory management of anti-aggregated and anticoagulated patients, with a special part in hip fracture surgery.

So, a wide scope of the topic was made with a great effort from all the authors and the invaluable support from Springer. I want to thank all of them for their confidence, aid, hard work, time (much time), exciting recommendations, and final result.

We hope this book will aid all of us in our daily practice, and, perhaps, the patients could benefit of our wish as doctors: to give them the best to improve their health as much as possible.

Juan V. Llau, M.D., Ph.D.
Editor

Contents

Contributors

José Aguirre, M.D. Division of Anesthesiology, Balgrist University Hospital, Zürich, Switzerland

Juan I. Arcelus, M.D., Ph.D. Department of Surgery, Hospital Universitario Virgen de las Nieves, University of Granada, Granada, Spain

Alain Borgeat, M.D. Division of Anesthesiology, Balgrist University Hospital, Zürich, Switzerland

Esther Ciércoles, M.D. Anaesthesia Department, Hospital Universitari Vall d'Hebron, Barcelona, Spain

Maria J. Colomina, M.D., Ph.D. Anaesthesia Department, Hospital Universitari Vall d'Hebron, Barcelona, Spain

Raquel Ferrandis, M.D., Ph.D. Department of Anaesthesiology and Critical Care, Hospital Clinic Universitari de València, Valencia, Spain

Human Physiology Department, School of Medicine, Valencia University, Valencia, Spain

Ola E. Dahl, M.D., DocMedsci Department of Medical Science, Innlandet Hospital Trust, Centre of Medical Science, Education and Innovation, Brumunddal, Norway

Thrombosis Research Institute, Chelsea, London, UK

Bengt I. Eriksson, M.D., Ph.D. Orthopaedic Department, Surgical Sciences, University of Gothenburg, Mölndal, Sweden

Department of Orthopaedic Surgery, SU/Molndal, Mölndal, Sweden

Steven E. Flores, M.D. Department of Orthopedic Surgery, University of Texas Health Science Center at Houston, Houston, TX, USA

Ajay K. Kakkar, M.B.B.S., Ph.D. Department of Surgery,
University College London, London, UK

University College London Hospitals NHS Foundation Trust, London, UK

Thrombosis Research Institute, Chelsea, London, UK

Sibylle A. Kozek-Langenecker, M.D., Professor M.B.A. Department of
Anesthesiology and Intensive Care, Evangelic Hospital Vienna, Vienna, Austria

Lasse J. Lapidus, M.D., Ph.D. Department of Clinical Science and Education,
Karolinska Institutet, Södersjukhuset Hospital, Stockholm, Stockholm, Sweden

Department of Orthopedics, Karolinska Institutet, Södersjukhuset Hospital,
Stockholm, Stockholm, Sweden

Juan V. Llau, M.D., Ph.D. Department of Anesthesiology and Critical Care,
Hospital Clinico Universitario, Valencia, Spain

Human Physiology and Anaesthesiology, School of Medicine,
Catholic University "San Vincente Martir", Valencia, Spain

Walter R. Lowe, M.D. Department of Orthopedic Surgery,
University of Texas Health Science Center at Houston, Houston, TX, USA

Memorial Hermann Sports Medicine Clinic, Houston, TX, USA

Manuel Monreal, M.D., Ph.D. Department of Internal Medicine,
Hospital Germans Trias I Pujol, Badalona, Barcelona, Spain

Lidia Mora, M.D. Anaesthesia Department,
Hospital Universitari Vall d'Hebron, Barcelona, Spain

James E. Muntz, M.D., FACP Medicine and Orthopedics Departments,
Baylor College of Medicine, Houston, TX, USA

Memorial Hermann Sports Medicine Clinic, Houston, TX, USA

Sophie K. Rushton-Smith, B.Sc., Ph.D. Thrombosis Research Institute, Chelsea,
London, UK

David J. Warwick, M.D., FRCS, FRCS (Orth) Department of Orthopaedic
Surgery, University of Southampton, Southampton, UK

Chapter 1
Thromboembolism in Orthopedic Surgery: Scope of the Problem

Bengt I. Eriksson and Ola E. Dahl

Abstract Major surgery or traumas of the lower extremities trigger the coagulation cascade, and the physiologic equilibrium between factors promoting and retarding coagulation is disturbed resulting in a hypercoagulable state. In these patients, a reduced venous flow and impaired endothelial function further increase the risk of developing deep-vein thrombosis and pulmonary embolism. Pulmonary embolism is estimated to contribute to half of all perioperative mortality after major orthopedic surgery in unprotected patients, and deep-vein thrombosis is the main source of pulmonary emboli.

Keywords Thromboembolism • Orthopedic surgery • Antithrombotic drugs

Introduction

Major surgery or traumas of the lower extremities trigger the coagulation cascade and the physiologic equilibrium between factors promoting, and retarding coagulation is disturbed resulting in a hypercoagulable state. In these patients, a reduced venous flow and impaired endothelial function further increase the risk of developing deep-vein thrombosis and pulmonary embolism. Pulmonary embolism is estimated to contribute to half of all perioperative mortality after major orthopedic surgery in unprotected patients, and deep-vein thrombosis is the main source of pulmonary emboli [1].

B.I. Eriksson, M.D., Ph.D. (✉)
Department of Orthopaedic Surgery, SU/Molndal,
SE-43180 Molndal, Sweden

Orthopaedic Department,
Surgical Sciences, University of Gothenburg, Molndal, Sweden
e-mail: b.eriksson@orthop.gu.se

O.E. Dahl, M.D., DocMedsci
Department of Medical Science, Innlandet Hospital Trust, Centre of Medical Science,
Education and Innovation, Brumunddal, Norway

Thrombosis Research Institute, Chelsea, London, UK
e-mail: oladahl@start.no

J.V. Llau (ed.), *Thromboembolism in Orthopedic Surgery*,
DOI 10.1007/978-1-4471-4336-9_1, © Springer-Verlag London 2013

Background

Deep-vein thrombosis (DVT) and pulmonary embolism (PE) are serious and potentially fatal complications after major orthopedic surgery. In a large overview of controlled trials, Collins and coworkers [1] demonstrated a clear benefit of low-dose unfractionated heparin (UFH) in major orthopedic, general, and urologic surgery, reducing both fatal pulmonary embolism and deep-vein thrombosis. Since Sevitt and Gallagher [2] first demonstrated the advantages of thromboprophylaxis, many different prophylactic methods, both mechanical and chemical, have been described. Chemical methods include the use of different anticoagulants, such as low-dose UFH, low-molecular-weight heparin (LMWH), specific factor Xa inhibitors, specific thrombin inhibitors, vitamin K antagonists (VKAs), or platelet inhibitors. Mechanical techniques involve the use of graduated, elastic compression stockings, or different modalities of lower extremity pumping systems.

Chemical Thromboprophylaxis

In a very early controlled study, Sevitt and Gallagher [2] published a report on 300 patients undergoing hip fracture surgery, comparing phenindione with no treatment, and they could demonstrate 80 % reduction of fatal pulmonary embolism with anticoagulant treatment. In 1977, Charnley and coworkers published a 12-year material of 7,959 patients undergoing total hip arthroplasty showing that pulmonary embolism was the largest single cause of death [3]. At the start of their registration, 15.2 % nonfatal and 2.3 % fatal PE was found. As a consequence of the high rate of venous embolism in their department, they introduced pharmacological antithrombotic treatment. Initially, it caused frequent bleeding complications, but after several years of trial and error, they found an acceptable regimen and the rate of PE was reduced by 50 %. Based on their experience, they recommended colleagues to use general chemical thromboprophylaxis in this clinical setting.

During the same period as Charnley and his group published their data, two other randomized clinical trials were published. One trial by VV Kakkar and colleagues [4, 5] and one by Kline and associates [6]. Both groups showed similar results, i.e., chemoprophylaxis (UFH and Dextran70) significantly reduced autopsy verified fatal PE in surgical patients. In other words, the benefit of chemical prophylaxis had clearly been demonstrated, and it was calculated that 7 lives were saved for each 1,000 patients undergoing surgery [4], thus there was no doubt that this was a substantial improvement in the prevention of severe postsurgical complications. Collins and coworkers [1] reviewed 74 controlled studies on different types of surgery, including 12 randomized studies on patients undergoing elective total hip arthroplasty, and they reported a DVT rate of 46 % in screened unprotected patients, and the incidence of fatal PE was 1.6 %. This meta-analysis demonstrated a relative reduction of the DVT rate by 50 % when UFH was administered and the incidence of PE, including fatal PE, was reduced correspondingly. Because of these serious complications in unprotected patients, routine prophylaxis after major orthopedic surgery has been recommended.

Surgeons are concerned about complications associated with the use of anticoagulants, particularly bleeding [4, 7]. However, there is extensive data from both meta-analyzes and randomized clinical studies that there is limited increase in the rate of clinically important bleeding complications when optimal regimens of either UFH, LMWH, or VKA are implemented [1, 8–13].

In 1986, Turpie et al. performed a randomized placebo-controlled trial demonstrating that LMWH was effective and safe in patients undergoing elective hip surgery, and they also showed that prophylactic treatment could be started postoperatively [14]. LMWHs gradually replaced UFH after early reports from several research groups [15, 16], and in a meta-analysis, Nurmohamed et al. could demonstrate that LMWH was preferable to unfractionated heparin in the prevention of deep-vein thrombosis and pulmonary embolism in patients undergoing major orthopedic surgery [9].

A large progress was achieved when LMWHs were introduced, and once (or twice) daily administration implied more convenient out-of-hospital prophylaxis of thromboembolism. Moreover, LMWH did not require routine monitoring or dose adjustment, which facilitated ambulatory treatment of deep-vein thrombosis and pulmonary embolism. Heparin-induced thrombocytopenia (HIT) was a feared complication with UFH, and this was less frequently seen with the LMWHs [17].

Smaller fractions of the active part of the heparin molecule were also presented in the market, e.g., fondaparinux. This small molecule was seemingly a more effective chemical than the larger heparin chains but became associated with an increased risk of bleeding. Postmarketing reports to European medicines agency (EMA) recently showed a higher rate of serious bleedings with fondaparinux than with the LMWHs [18]. Consequently, EMA recommended a lower dose in particular in elderly and those with reduced renal function.

Warfarin was the only available oral anticoagulant until recently when a break through was reached and several new oral formulations were developed, e.g., (xi) melagatran, dabigatran, rivaroxaban, and apixaban, of which (xi)melagatran was withdrawn from the market due to liver toxicity. Since the new oral anticoagulants do not need any routine monitoring, they offer substantial out-of-hospital benefits as compared to VKAs and the parenterally administered heparin derivatives. Antiplatelet drugs, mainly acetylsalicylic acid, do not seem to have sufficient efficacy and are not recommended as a sole prophylactic regimen [19].

Mechanical Devices

Specially designed elastic stockings have been developed enhancing increased blood flow in the deep veins. In general surgical patients, graduated elastic stockings might add a positive effect in combination with UFH or LMWH, reducing the rate of DVT. However, such an additive effect seems to be difficult to detect in patients undergoing hip or knee arthroplasty. Today, most of the graduated elastic stockings are used to limit edema after surgery. Mechanical devices like foot pumps and other pneumatic compression devices have shown conflicting results and compliance [20]. Application and removal may be cumbersome, and 24-h a day use is problematic without assistance by educated health personal. Mechanical devices could, however, be feasible in cases when chemical thromboprophylaxis is temporarily or permanently contraindicated.

End Points and Diagnostic Methodology in Antithrombotic Trials

Development of new and more effective anticoagulant drugs has been in focus for many years. Initially, trial end points were clinical DVT and autopsy-verified PE. In the modern health care system, it has, however, been increasingly difficult to use these end points due to many different reasons, e.g., more effective postoperative mobilization and physiotherapy in combination with more effective antithrombotic compounds have reduced the incidence of thromboembolic events markedly, hence surrogate end points including asymptomatic DVT have been introduced in clinical trials. Many surveillance methods have been used to identify DVT, but venography has been shown to be superior to other techniques [21]. In their meta-analysis of controlled clinical trials, Collins and coworkers could demonstrate a clear relationship between the reduction of total VTE and PE, and this has also been shown in more recent meta-analyzes comparing long-duration versus short-term VTE prophylaxis after total hip arthroplasty [22–24]. This is the rationale behind the composite end point of total VTE, combining the incidence of thrombi both in the distal and proximal region together with PE and total mortality. There is, however, some variation in the definition of efficacy end points in different trials, and moreover, there is a considerable variation in venographic technique and assessment criteria in different studies [25]. For this reason, a direct comparison of absolute DVT rates in different trials is almost impossible. Regarding safety results, the difference in definitions of bleeding is even more complex, which makes comparisons between trials more or less meaningless. Thus, if a new antithrombotic regimen may seem favorable versus another compound, such an assumption may not necessarily be correct. It can only be assessed in head-to-head trials of the two compounds. However, conduction of such trials sponsored by pharmaceutical industry is unlikely to be performed within the near future (Dahl, personal communication 2010).

Systemic Thromboembolic Events

In recent years, it has become more and more evident that arterial and venous thromboembolic events may share some comorbid characteristics predisposing to systemic thromboembolic events, especially when the haemostatic system is triggered.

Orthopedic trauma and surgery induce a massive thrombin generation and cellular activation that affect both the venous and arterial side. This may lead to thromboembolic manifestations from several organs and from mild to serious complications like respiratory distress, stroke, retinal vein thrombosis, angina, myocardial infarction, deep-vein thrombosis, and pulmonary embolism. These events may appear from the time of surgery and a long time after the operation due to cellular and chemical crosstalk between hemostasis and inflammation. Thrombin is the key regulator of this process. Procoagulant debris from the damaged bone marrow, conjugates of activated cells and microparticles flow with the venous blood and reach the arterial circulation through several routes. In the lung vessels, activated blood cells may adhere to the endothelium and entrap, causing shunt effects, drop in oxygen tension, and respiratory distress. In addition, about 30 % of the population have a patent foramen ovale. Through all these vessel shunts, activated cells and cell fragments may pass over to the arterial side and be distributed with the blood stream to end organs or accumulate in atherosclerotic arteries and contribute to arterial complications.

Initiation of Prophylaxis and Regimens of Antithrombotic Compounds

The optimal dose level and timing of different antithrombotics in relation to specific surgical procedures are titrated in several trial programs unique for each compound [19]. However, in these trials, mainly healthy patients are enrolled, and the regimens and recommendations based on these results are to be transferred into clinical practice which often is more complex since patients with many different comorbidities require special care. Of practical importance is also that antithrombotic regimens need to be flexible regarding logistic difficulties, e.g., very short hospital stay or ambulatory care. There are a number of issues that have to be considered to adapt and tailor preventive regimens to different clinical settings, populations, and individuals.

Duration of Thromboprophylaxis

After many years of in-hospital thromboprophylaxis, Scurr and associates started several years ago to investigate whether there was a continued risk of developing thrombi in the weeks following surgery. Patients undergoing abdominal surgery were followed with multiple fibrinogen scanning technique, and in 25 % of the cases, fresh thrombi were demonstrated between 1 and 6 weeks after surgery [26]. This initiated an intense debate and demand for more studies also in orthopedic patients known for their high rate of venous thromboembolism. During the 1990s, several 4–5 weeks out-of-hospital placebo-controlled surveillance trials were conducted with mandatory venography [23, 27–31]. These studies showed that the prevalence and incidence of deep-vein thromboses continued to accumulate after hospital discharge during the study intervals. Continuation of LMWH prophylaxis during the entire study periods reduced risk of developing symptomatic deep-vein thromboses with two thirds. However, we have to consider the delicate balance between antithrombotic effect and bleeding, which is of special importance when potent antithrombotic chemicals are used perioperatively or in long duration out-of-hospital treatment [32]. In elderly patients and those with reduced renal function, there is also a potential risk of drug accumulation, both with low-molecular-weight heparins and many of the new oral anticoagulants.

Reduced Incidence of Postoperative Venous Thromboembolism

During the last two decades, more efficacious antithrombotic drugs have been introduced but also improved anesthetic and surgical techniques allowing early mobilization and accelerated rehabilitation, all of which most probably have contributed to a reduction in thromboembolic complications [33].

Long-Term Clinical Course of Venous Thromboembolic Conditions

After the first event of deep-vein thrombosis, recurrence is seen in up to 30 %. This increases the risk of six-folds of developing venous insufficiency and postphlebitic syndrome. Up to 30 % of patients with deep-vein thrombosis may experience this condition within 5 years of which 7 % are so severe that it causes permanent disability and substantial costs on regional health budgets. This syndrome consists of leg swelling, discomfort, skin changes and ulceration [34]. Chronic pulmonary hypertension is a common sequelae after the first episode of pulmonary embolism. One out of 25 will suffer from life-long respiratory and cardiac insufficiency that will disable the patients [35].

Contraindications to Anticoagulant Treatment

Even if the benefit with antithrombotic prophylactic therapy outweighs the harm, we have to remember the relative and absolute contraindications to anticoagulant treatment. Absolute contraindications include active hemorrhage and unstable conditions with multiple injuries. Relative contraindications include patients with an active intracranial lesion, a previous history of cerebral or gastrointestinal hemorrhage, and of course all patients with an increased risk of bleeding. If there is a history of abnormal bleeding events or fresh trauma, thromboprophylaxis with mechanical methods may be considered.

Future Directions and Conclusions

Emerging oral anticoagulants in advanced clinical development have important advantages over VKAs, including a rapid onset of action, a predictable anticoagulant effects that minimize the need for routine coagulation monitoring and a low propensity for drug or dietary interactions. The superior pharmacological properties and convenience of the new oral anticoagulants compared with existing anticoagulants have translated into improvements in efficacy and safety in initial randomized trials. Dabigatran, rivaroxaban, and apixaban are the agents most advanced in development. Several other new oral anticoagulants will also likely reach the market over the next few years and thereby improve the management of thromboembolic disorders. Recognition that bleeding is associated with adverse outcomes in patients with cardiovascular disease and concern about the lack of antidotes has focused attention on the risk of bleeding with all of the new oral anticoagulants. In particular, the potential bleeding risks incurred by combining some of the specific platelet aggregation inhibitors with the new oral anticoagulants will require further evaluation. Key characteristics include their renal elimination, which is of particular importance in elderly patients and in those with renal dysfunction. Although speculation still remains regarding the optimal target of anticoagulants (inhibition of FIIa or FXa, etc.), the pharmacokinetic characteristics, dosing strategies, and side effects may be more clinically relevant. Of practical importance is that thromboprophylaxis needs to be robust regarding logistic difficulties, e.g., very short hospital stay or ambulatory care. There are a number of issues that have to be considered to adapt and even tailor preventative regimens to different clinical settings, populations, and individuals.

References

1. Collins R, Scrimgeour A, Yusuf S, et al. Reduction in fatal pulmonary embolism and venous thrombosis by perioperative administration of subcutaneous heparin: overview of results of randomized trials in general, orthopedic, and urology surgery. N Engl J Med. 1988;318: 1162–73.
2. Sevitt S, Gallagher NG. Prevention of venous thrombosis and pulmonary embolism in injured patients: a trial of anticoagulant prophylaxis with phenindione in middle-aged and elderly patients with fractured necks of femur. Lancet. 1959;2:981–9.
3. Johnson R, Green JR, Charnley J. Pulmonary embolism and its prophylaxis following the Charnley total hip replacement. Clin Orthop Relat Res. 1977;127:123–32.
4. Anonymous. Prevention of fatal postoperative pulmonary embolism by low doses of heparin. An international multicentre trial coordinated by Kakkar VV, Corrigan TP and Fossard DP. Lancet. 1975;2(7924):45–51.
5. Kakkar VV, Corrigan TP, Fossard DP, et al. Prevention of fatal postoperative pulmonary embolism by low doses of heparin. Reappraisal of results of international multicentre trial. Lancet. 1977;1(8011):567–9.
6. Kline A, Hughes LE, Campbell H, et al. Dextran 70 in prophylaxis of thromboembolic disease after surgery: a clinically oriented randomized double-blind trial. BMJ. 1975;2:109–12.

7. van Ooijen B. Subcutaneous heparin and postoperative wound hematomas: a prospective, double-blind, randomised study. Arch Surg. 1986;121:937–40.
8. Clagett GP, Reisch JS. Prevention of venous thromboembolism in general surgical patients: results of meta-analysis. Ann Surg. 1988;208:227–40.
9. Nurmohamed MT, Rosendaal FR, Buller HR, et al. Low-molecular-weight heparin versus standard heparin in general and orthopaedic surgery: a meta-analysis. Lancet. 1992;340:152–6.
10. Kakkar VV, Cohen AT, Edmonson RA, et al. Low molecular weight versus standard heparin for prevention of venous thromboembolism after major abdominal surgery. Lancet. 1993; 341:259–65.
11. Jorgensen LN, Wille-Jorgensen P, Hauch O. Prophylaxis of postoperative thromboembolism with low molecular weight heparins. Br J Surg. 1993;80:689–704.
12. Thomas DP. Does low molecular weight heparin cause less bleeding? Thromb Haemost. 1997;78:1422–5.
13. Koch A, Ziegler S, Breitschwerdt H, et al. Low molecular weight heparin and unfractionated heparin in thrombosis prophylaxis: meta-analysis based on original patient data. Thromb Res. 2001;102:295–309.
14. Turpie AG, Levine MN, Hirsh J, et al. A randomized controlled trial of a low-molecular-weight heparin (enoxaparin) to prevent deep-vein thrombosis in patients undergoing elective hip surgery. N Engl J Med. 1986;315(15):925–9.
15. Bergqvist D, Mätzsch T, Burmark US, et al. Low molecular weight heparin given the evening before surgery compared with conventional low-dose heparin in prevention of thrombosis. Br J Surg. 1988;75(9):888–91.
16. Eriksson BI, Zachrisson BE, Teger-Nilsson AC, et al. Thrombosis prophylaxis with low molecular weight heparin in total hip replacement. Br J Surg. 1988;75(11):1053–7.
17. Monreal M, Lafoz E, Olive A, et al. Comparison of subcutaneous unfractionated heparin with a low molecular weight heparin (Fragmin) in patients with venous thromboembolism and contraindications to coumarin. Thromb Haemost. 1994;71:7–11.
18. European Medicines Agency. Fondaparinux summary of product characteristics. 2007. http:// www.ema.europa.eu/docs/en_GB/document_library/EPAR__Product_Information/ human/000403/WC500027746.pdf. Accessed 16 Sep 2010.
19. Geerts WH, Bergqvist D, Pineo GF, et al. Prevention of venous thromboembolism. Chest. 2008;133:381S–453.
20. Warwick D, Harrison J, Glew D, et al. Comparison of the use of a foot pump with the use of low-molecular-weight heparin for the prevention of deep-vein-thrombosis after total hip replacement. A prospective randomized trial. J Bone Joint Surg Am. 1998;80:1158–86.
21. Schellong SM, Beyer J, Kakkar AK, et al. Ultrasound screening for asymptomatic deep vein thrombosis after major orthopaedic surgery: the VENUS study. J Thromb Haemost. 2007;5: 1431–7.
22. Eikelboom JW, Quinlan DJ, Douketis JD. Extended duration prophylaxis against venous thromboembolism after total hip or knee replacement: a meta-analysis of the randomised trials. Lancet. 2001;358:9–15.
23. Hull RD, Pineo GF, Stein PD, et al. Extended out-of hospital low-molecular-weight heparin prophylaxis against deep venous thrombosis in patients after elective hip arthroplasty: a systematic review. Ann Intern Med. 2001;135:858–69.
24. Cohen AT, Bailey CS, Alikhan R, et al. Extended thromboprophylaxis with low molecular weight heparin reduces symptomatic venous thromboembolism following lower limb arthroplasty: a meta-analysis. Thromb Haemost. 2001;85:940–1.
25. Quinlan DJ, Eikelboom JW, Dahl OE, et al. Association between asymptomatic deep vein thrombosis detected by venography and symptomatic venous thromboembolism in patients undergoing elective hip or knee surgery. J Thromb Haemost. 2007;5:1438–43.
26. Scurr JH, et al. Deep venous thrombosis: a continuing problem. BMJ. 1988;297(6640):28.
27. Planes A, Vochelle N, Darmon JY, et al. Risk of deep-venous thrombosis after discharge in patients having undergone total hip replacement; double-blind randomised comparison of enoxaparin versus placebo. Lancet. 1996;348:224–8.

28. Bergqvist D, Benoni G, Bjørgell O, et al. Low-molecular-weight heparin (enoxaparin) as prophylaxis against venous thromboembolism after total hip replacement. N Engl J Med. 1996;5:696–700.
29. Dahl OE, et al. Prolonged thromboprophylaxis following hip replacement surgery;-results of a double-blind, prospective, randomised, placebo-controlled study with dalteparin (Fragmin). Thromb Haemost. 1997;77:26–31.
30. Lassen MR, Borris LC, Anderson BS, et al. Efficacy and safety of prolonged thromboprophylaxis with a low molecular weight heparin (dalteparin) after total hip arthroplasty the Danish Prolonged Prophylaxis (DaPP) Study. Thromb Res. 1998;89:281–7.
31. Comp PC, Spiro TE, Friedman RJ, et al. Prolonged enoxaparin therapy to prevent venous thromboembolism after primary hip or knee replacement. J Bone Joint Surg Am. 2001;83: 336–45.
32. Dahl OE, Quinlan DJ, Eikelboom J, et al. A critical appraisal of bleeding events reported in venous thromboembolism prevention trials of patients undergoing hip and knee arthroplasty. J Thromb Haemost. 2010;8:1966–75.
33. Bjørnarå BT, Gudmundsen TE, Dahl OE. Frequency and timing of clinical venous thromboembolism after major joint surgery. J Bone Joint Surg Br. 2006;88(3):386–91.
34. Prandoni P, Villalta S, Bagatella P, et al. The clinical course of deep-vein thrombosis. Prospective long-term follow-up of 528 symptomatic patients. Haematologica. 1997;82: 423–8.
35. Pengo V, Lensing AW, Prins MH, et al. Incidence of chronic thromboembolic pulmonary hypertension after pulmonary embolism. N Engl J Med. 2004;350:2257–64.

Chapter 2
Incidence of Venous Thromboembolism in Orthopedic Surgery

Ajay K. Kakkar and Sophie K. Rushton-Smith

Abstract Venous thromboembolic disease in hospitalized patients results in substantial mortality, morbidity, and healthcare resource use. While the true incidence of venous thromboembolism (VTE) is difficult to determine, autopsy studies have shown that 5–10 % of hospital deaths are attributable to pulmonary embolism. Major orthopedic surgery is associated with a very high risk of VTE: without thromboprophylaxis objectively confirmed deep-vein thrombosis may occur in up to 60 % of patients within 2 weeks after lower extremity orthopedic surgery. Between 10 and 30 % of symptomatic VTE events present as proximal deep-vein thrombosis, with the potential to lead to post-thrombotic syndrome or pulmonary embolism. As both symptomatic and subclinical thromboembolism are common in patients undergoing major orthopedic surgery, risk assessment and, where appropriate, thromboprophylaxis should be considered.

Keywords Deep-vein thrombosis • Incidence • Orthopedic surgery • Pulmonary embolism • Venous thromboembolism

Introduction

Venous thromboembolic disease in hospitalized patients is an important healthcare concern, resulting in significant mortality, morbidity, and healthcare resource expenditure. Over 40 years ago, Kakkar et al. [1, 2] determined the frequency of venous

A.K. Kakkar, M.B.B.S., Ph.D. (✉)
Department of Surgery, University College London, London, UK

University College London Hospitals NHS Foundation Trust, London, UK

Thrombosis Research Institute, Manresa Road,
Emmanuel Kaye Building, Chelsea, London SW3 6LR, UK
e-mail: akkakkar@tri-london.ac.uk

S.K. Rushton-Smith, B.Sc., Ph.D.
Thrombosis Research Institute, Manresa Road,
Emmanuel Kaye Building, Chelsea, London SW3 6LR, UK
e-mail: srushton-smith@tri-london.ac.uk

J.V. Llau (ed.), *Thromboembolism in Orthopedic Surgery*,
DOI 10.1007/978-1-4471-4336-9_2, © Springer-Verlag London 2013

thrombosis in general surgical patients using I^{125} labeled fibrinogen leg scanning and were thus able to describe the natural history of postoperative deep-vein thrombosis (DVT). Better understanding of the natural history and the course of venous thromboembolism (VTE) and its associated risk factors has led to strategies for identifying individuals at risk of VTE in the perioperative period, together with methods of quantifying that risk, and approaches for the prevention of thrombotic episodes.

While many patients with a thrombosis remain asymptomatic and the thrombi resolve without causing complications, some patients will develop symptomatic DVT or pulmonary embolism, whereas others will suffer a fatal pulmonary embolism as the first manifestation of their thrombosis [3]. Approximately eight in ten patients who develop pulmonary emboli will have no evidence of peripheral venous thrombosis before presenting with pulmonary embolism [4].

The long-term sequelae of VTE also present a considerable healthcare concern and include post-thrombotic syndrome – a chronic, potentially disabling condition – recurrent VTE, and chronic pulmonary hypertension [5–9].

The aim of this chapter is to present and discuss the frequency of VTE events among patients undergoing orthopedic surgery.

Determining the Incidence of Venous Thromboembolism

The true incidence of VTE and its associated morbidity and mortality is difficult to determine. Often, VTE is clinically silent, signs and symptoms are non-specific, and screening tests are not always sufficiently sensitive to detect disease in asymptomatic patients. The reported rates of VTE show considerable variation for a variety of reasons, some examples of which are given in Table 2.1.

Autopsy studies, which are increasingly infrequent nowadays, have shown that between 5 and 10 % of hospital deaths are attributable to pulmonary embolism [16–19]. Pulmonary embolism is therefore widely reported to be the most common cause of preventable death in patients hospitalized for surgical procedures [20].

Table 2.1 Potential reasons for variation in reported rates of VTE [10–15]

Distribution of risk factors (e.g., age, lifestyle factors)

Geographic differences (e.g., age, general health and nutritional state, socio-economic status, genetic, or environmental factors)

Variations in patient management or surgical technique (e.g., duration of surgery, length of hospitalization, period of immobilization, type of prosthesis, unilateral vs. bilateral)

Fluctuations over time (e.g., variations in surgical technique, use of prophylaxis)

Methods of diagnosis (e.g., I^{125}-fibrinogen uptake test, venography)

Type of anesthesia used (e.g., regional, general)

Use and type of thromboprophylaxis (e.g., mechanical, pharmacological)

Duration of follow-up/timing of diagnostic end point

Study type (e.g., autopsy, clinical trial, observational study)

Representativeness of the population

Statistical reasons (e.g., small study sizes, leading to wide confidence intervals)

Recent data on the frequency of VTE in surgical patients in the absence of prophylaxis are rare because few contemporary studies include untreated control groups.

Orthopedic Surgery and Thrombosis

Major orthopedic surgery, which includes total hip replacement (THR), total knee replacement (TKR), and hip fracture surgery, is associated with a very high risk of postoperative VTE [21]. The level of VTE risk associated with surgery depends upon a combination of patient-specific predisposing factors and factors associated with the surgical procedure itself [22–24] (see Chap. 4). In terms of Virchow's triad of contributing factors for thrombus formation, the risk of postoperative VTE relates to perioperative immobilization, activated coagulation, and transient depression of fibrinolysis.

Without thromboprophylaxis, the rates of objectively confirmed DVT occurring within 7–14 days after lower extremity orthopedic surgery are around 40–60 % [21, 22]. Most of these thrombi resolve spontaneously, but a small percentage (1–14 %) will progress to symptomatic VTE [12, 25–34], often presenting after the patient has been discharged from the hospital [35–37].

Between 10 and 30 % of symptomatic VTE events present as proximal DVT [22]. This is a clinically more important manifestation than distal DVT because it is more frequently associated with post-thrombotic syndrome and has greater potential to embolize and cause pulmonary embolism [21, 38–40].

Total Knee Replacement

Without thromboprophylaxis, the reported risk of venographically documented DVT in patients undergoing TKR ranges from 41 to 85 % [22]. The rate of proximal DVT, as a thrombus extension from the calf veins to the popliteal or femoral veins, varies from 5 to 22 % [22].

Limited data are available on the incidence of pulmonary embolism after TKR in patients not given thromboprophylaxis. In two studies in which the objective end point included the diagnosis of pulmonary embolism on a perfusion lung scan, 22 % of 186 patients and 33 % of 12 patients showed symptoms of pulmonary embolism [15, 41]. The rates of symptomatic pulmonary embolism following TKR without prophylaxis are much lower, ranging from 1 to 2 %, and that of fatal pulmonary embolism is <1 % [11, 42].

Total Hip Replacement

THR is a common procedure, which is being performed with increasing frequency in elderly patients [43]. In the absence of thromboprophylaxis, the risk of venographically documented DVT in patients undergoing THR ranges from 42 to 57 % and from 2 to 5 % for symptomatic events [22, 39, 44, 45]. While these rates are lower than those reported for TKR, perhaps due to the use of a tourniquet during knee replacement surgery [46], the risk of the more clinically important proximal DVT is higher, at 18–36 % [22, 39, 44, 45, 47–54]. The rate of symptomatic VTE in untreated patients is 2–5 % and that of fatal pulmonary embolism is 0.33 % [21].

The risk of VTE extends beyond the period of hospitalization, as shown in a study of 179 patients undergoing THR who were without venogram-proven DVT at hospital discharge [37]. In this study, 20 % of the patients given placebo developed venographic evidence of DVT compared with 7.1 % of patients randomized to enoxaparin prophylaxis [37]. VTE is also reported to be the most frequent cause for hospital readmission following THR surgery [55].

Hip Fracture Surgery

Patients undergoing hip fracture surgery are at very high risk of VTE. Thrombotic disease is a common cause of mortality and morbidity in this population. Among these patients, 46–60 % have venographic evidence of DVT, with 23–30 % of cases involving the proximal veins [22]. Even with the benefit of prophylaxis, symptomatic, objectively confirmed VTE has been reported to occur within 3 months of surgery in 1.3–8.2 % of this population [21, 56]. In a retrospective study of 470 patients treated for hip fractures who were not given thromboprophylaxis, the overall mortality rate within 1 month of the fracture was 18.5 % [57]; 19.5 % of these patients were found on autopsy to have died from pulmonary embolism.

Conclusion

Both symptomatic and subclinical thromboembolism are common in patients undergoing major orthopedic surgery. In view of the unpredictable nature of their complication, risk assessment and – where appropriate – thromboprophylaxis should be considered.

References

1. Kakkar VV, Howe CT, Flanc C, et al. Natural history of postoperative deep-vein thrombosis. Lancet. 1969;2(7614):230–2.
2. Kakkar V. The diagnosis of deep vein thrombosis using the 125I fibrinogen test. Arch Surg. 1972;104:152–9.
3. Lindblad B, Eriksson A, Bergqvist D. Autopsy-verified pulmonary embolism in a surgical department: analysis of the period from 1951 to 1988. Br J Surg. 1991;78(7):849–52.

4. Stein PD, Henry JW. Prevalence of acute pulmonary embolism among patients in a general hospital and at autopsy. Chest. 1995;108(4):978–81.
5. Prandoni P, Lensing AW, Cogo A, et al. The long-term clinical course of acute deep venous thrombosis. Ann Intern Med. 1996;125(1):1–7.
6. Cushman M, Tsai AW, White RH, et al. Deep vein thrombosis and pulmonary embolism in two cohorts: the longitudinal investigation of thromboembolism etiology. Am J Med. 2004;117(1): 19–25.
7. Heit JA, Mohr DN, Silverstein MD, et al. Predictors of recurrence after deep vein thrombosis and pulmonary embolism: a population-based cohort study. Arch Intern Med. 2000;160(6): 761–8.
8. Mohr DN, Silverstein MD, Heit JA, et al. The venous stasis syndrome after deep venous thrombosis or pulmonary embolism: a population-based study. Mayo Clin Proc. 2000;75(12): 1249–56.
9. McColl MD, Ellison J, Greer IA, et al. Prevalence of the post-thrombotic syndrome in young women with previous venous thromboembolism. Br J Haematol. 2000;108(2):272–4.
10. Lynch AF, Bourne RB, Rorabeck CH, et al. Deep-vein thrombosis and continuous passive motion after total knee arthroplasty. J Bone Joint Surg Am. 1988;70(1):11–4.
11. Stringer MD, Steadman CA, Hedges AR, et al. Deep vein thrombosis after elective knee surgery. An incidence study in 312 patients. J Bone Joint Surg Br. 1989;71(3):492–7.
12. Stulberg BN, Insall JN, Williams GW, et al. Deep-vein thrombosis following total knee replacement. An analysis of six hundred and thirty-eight arthroplasties. J Bone Joint Surg Am. 1984;66(2):194–201.
13. Haas SB, Insall JN, Scuderi GR, et al. Pneumatic sequential-compression boots compared with aspirin prophylaxis of deep-vein thrombosis after total knee arthroplasty. J Bone Joint Surg Am. 1990;72(1):27–31.
14. Lotke PA, Ecker ML, Alavi A, et al. Indications for the treatment of deep venous thrombosis following total knee replacement. J Bone Joint Surg Am. 1984;66(2):202–8.
15. Lynch JA, Baker PL, Polly RE, et al. Mechanical measures in the prophylaxis of postoperative thromboembolism in total knee arthroplasty. Clin Orthop Relat Res. 1990;260:24–9.
16. Lindblad B, Sternby NH, Bergqvist D. Incidence of venous thromboembolism verified by necropsy over 30 years. BMJ. 1991;302(6778):709–11.
17. Sandler DA, Martin JF. Autopsy proven pulmonary embolism in hospital patients: are we detecting enough deep vein thrombosis? J R Soc Med. 1989;82(4):203–5.
18. Alikhan R, Peters F, Wilmott R, et al. Fatal pulmonary embolism in hospitalised patients: a necropsy review. J Clin Pathol. 2004;57(12):1254–7.
19. Hauch O, Jorgensen LN, Khattar SC, et al. Fatal pulmonary embolism associated with surgery. An autopsy study. Acta Chir Scand. 1990;156(11–12):747–9.
20. Goldhaber SZ, Turpie AG. Prevention of venous thromboembolism among hospitalized medical patients. Circulation. 2005;111(1):e1–3.
21. Geerts WH, Bergqvist D, Pineo GF, et al. Prevention of venous thromboembolism: American college of chest physicians evidence-based clinical practice guidelines (8th edition). Chest. 2008;133(6 Suppl):381S–453.
22. Geerts WH, Pineo GF, Heit JA, et al. Prevention of venous thromboembolism: the seventh ACCP conference on antithrombotic and thrombolytic therapy. Chest. 2004;126(3 Suppl):338S–400.
23. Heit JA, Silverstein MD, Mohr DN, et al. Risk factors for deep vein thrombosis and pulmonary embolism: a population-based case-control study. Arch Intern Med. 2000;160(6):809–15.
24. Heit JA, O'Fallon WM, Petterson TM, et al. Relative impact of risk factors for deep vein thrombosis and pulmonary embolism: a population-based study. Arch Intern Med. 2002;162(11):1245–8.
25. Ginsberg JS, Turkstra F, Buller HR, et al. Postthrombotic syndrome after hip or knee arthroplasty: a cross-sectional study. Arch Intern Med. 2000;160(5):669–72.
26. Kim YH, Oh SH, Kim JS. Incidence and natural history of deep-vein thrombosis after total hip arthroplasty. A prospective and randomised clinical study. J Bone Joint Surg Br. 2003;85(5): 661–5.

27. Collins R, Scrimgeour A, Yusuf S, et al. Reduction in fatal pulmonary embolism and venous thrombosis by perioperative administration of subcutaneous heparin. Overview of results of randomized trials in general, orthopedic, and urologic surgery. N Engl J Med. 1988;318(18): 1162–73.
28. Bergqvist D. Postoperative thromboembolism. New York: Springer; 1983.
29. Paiement GD, Bell D, Wessinger SJ, editors. New advances in the prevention, diagnosis, and cost effectiveness of venous thromboembolic disease in patients with total hip replacement. In: The hip, proceedings of the fourteenth open scientific meeting of the Hip Society, C.V. Mosby, Saint Louis, 1987, p. 94–119.
30. Leclerc JR, Gent M, Hirsh J, et al. The incidence of symptomatic venous thromboembolism after enoxaparin prophylaxis in lower extremity arthroplasty: a cohort study of 1,984 patients. Canadian Collaborative Group. Chest. 1998;114(2 Suppl Evidence):115S–8.
31. Dahl OE, Gudmundsen TE, Haukeland L. Late occurring clinical deep vein thrombosis in joint-operated patients. Acta Orthop Scand. 2000;71(1):47–50.
32. Colwell Jr CW, Collis DK, Paulson R, et al. Comparison of enoxaparin and warfarin for the prevention of venous thromboembolic disease after total hip arthroplasty. Evaluation during hospitalization and three months after discharge. J Bone Joint Surg Am. 1999;81(7):932–40.
33. Heit JA, Elliott CG, Trowbridge AA, et al. Ardeparin sodium for extended out-of-hospital prophylaxis against venous thromboembolism after total hip or knee replacement. A randomized, double-blind, placebo-controlled trial. Ann Intern Med. 2000;132(11):853–61.
34. Schiff RL, Kahn SR, Shrier I, et al. Identifying orthopedic patients at high risk for venous thromboembolism despite thromboprophylaxis. Chest. 2005;128(5):3364–71.
35. White RH, Romano PS, Zhou H, et al. Incidence and time course of thromboembolic outcomes following total hip or knee arthroplasty. Arch Intern Med. 1998;158(14):1525–31.
36. Warwick D, Friedman RJ, Agnelli G, et al. Insufficient duration of venous thromboembolism prophylaxis after total hip or knee replacement when compared with the time course of thromboembolic events: findings from the Global Orthopaedic Registry. J Bone Joint Surg Br. 2007;89(6):799–807.
37. Planes A, Vochelle N, Darmon JY, et al. Risk of deep-venous thrombosis after hospital discharge in patients having undergone total hip replacement: double-blind randomised comparison of enoxaparin versus placebo. Lancet. 1996;348(9022):224–8.
38. Kearon C. Natural history of venous thromboembolism. Semin Vasc Med. 2001;1(1):27–38.
39. Cordell-Smith JA, Williams SC, Harper WM, et al. Lower limb arthroplasty complicated by deep venous thrombosis. Prevalence and subjective outcome. J Bone Joint Surg Br. 2004; 86(1):99–101.
40. Pellegrini Jr VD, Donaldson CT, Farber DC, et al. The Mark Coventry Award: prevention of readmission for venous thromboembolism after total knee arthroplasty. Clin Orthop Relat Res. 2006;452:21–7.
41. McKenna R, Galante J, Bachmann F, et al. Prevention of venous thromboembolism after total knee replacement by high-dose aspirin or intermittent calf and thigh compression. Br Med J. 1980;280(6213):514–7.
42. Morrey BF, Adams RA, Ilstrup DM, et al. Complications and mortality associated with bilateral or unilateral total knee arthroplasty. J Bone Joint Surg Am. 1987;69(4):484–8.
43. Kurtz S, Ong K, Lau E, et al. Projections of primary and revision hip and knee arthroplasty in the United States from 2005 to 2030. J Bone Joint Surg Am. 2007;89(4):780–5.
44. Pellegrini Jr VD, Donaldson CT, Farber DC, et al. The John Charnley Award: prevention of readmission for venous thromboembolic disease after total hip arthroplasty. Clin Orthop Relat Res. 2005;441:56–62.
45. Lieberman JR, Hsu WK. Prevention of venous thromboembolic disease after total hip and knee arthroplasty. J Bone Joint Surg Am. 2005;87(9):2097–112.
46. Lijfering WM, van der Meer J. Pharmacological prevention of venous thromboembolism. In: van Beek JR, Buller HR, Oudkerk M, editors. Deep vein thrombosis and pulmonary embolism. Chichester: John Wiley and Sons, Ltd; 2009. p. 435–61.

47. Salvati EA, Pellegrini Jr VD, Sharrock NE, et al. Recent advances in venous thromboembolic prophylaxis during and after total hip replacement. J Bone Joint Surg Am. 2000;82(2): 252–70.
48. Phillips CB, Barrett JA, Losina E, et al. Incidence rates of dislocation, pulmonary embolism, and deep infection during the first six months after elective total hip replacement. J Bone Joint Surg Am. 2003;85-A(1):20–6.
49. Dahl OE, Caprini JA, Colwell Jr CW, et al. Fatal vascular outcomes following major orthopedic surgery. Thromb Haemost. 2005;93(5):860–6.
50. Howie C, Hughes H, Watts AC. Venous thromboembolism associated with hip and knee replacement over a ten-year period: a population-based study. J Bone Joint Surg Br. 2005;87(12): 1675–80.
51. Warwick D, Williams MH, Bannister GC. Death and thromboembolic disease after total hip replacement. A series of 1162 cases with no routine chemical prophylaxis. J Bone Joint Surg Br. 1995;77(1):6–10.
52. Fender D, Harper WM, Thompson JR, et al. Mortality and fatal pulmonary embolism after primary total hip replacement. Results from a regional hip register. J Bone Joint Surg Br. 1997;79(6):896–9.
53. Gillespie W, Murray D, Gregg PJ, et al. Risks and benefits of prophylaxis against venous thromboembolism in orthopaedic surgery. J Bone Joint Surg Br. 2000;82(4):475–9.
54. Turpie AG, Levine MN, Hirsh J, et al. A randomized controlled trial of a low-molecular-weight heparin (enoxaparin) to prevent deep-vein thrombosis in patients undergoing elective hip surgery. N Engl J Med. 1986;315(15):925–9.
55. Seagroatt V, Tan HS, Goldacre M, et al. Elective total hip replacement: incidence, emergency readmission rate, and postoperative mortality. BMJ. 1991;303(6815):1431–5.
56. Hitos K, Fletcher JP. Venous thromboembolism and fractured neck of femur. Thromb Haemost. 2005;94(5):991–6.
57. Riska EB. Incidence of thrombo-embolic disease in patients with hip fractures. Injury. 1970;2(2):155–8.

Chapter 3
Specific Risk Factors for Venous Thromboembolism in Orthopedics

Lasse J. Lapidus

Abstract Orthopedic surgery is a well-known risk factor for venous thromboembolism (VTE), especially hip and knee replacement but also fracture surgery in the lower limb. In the assessment of risk factors for specific procedures or injuries, it is important to remember the multifactorial etiology to VTE. In addition to the risk inherent to a specific clinical situation (e.g., specific injuries or specific surgical procedures), factors in the preoperative and postoperative setting can influence the risk for VTE. These include, for example, the type of anesthesia used, the use of tourniquet, and postoperative plaster cast immobilization. Also, a variety of patient characteristics such as high age, history of previous VTE, malignancy, and the use of oral contraceptives could increase the risk for VTE.

In this chapter, risk factors for VTE in specific orthopedic procedures and injuries are presented in detail.

Keywords Thrombosis • Risk factor • Orthopedic surgery • Injury • Prosthesis Fracture

Introduction

Venous thromboembolism (VTE) is a multifactorial disease where interactions between a large number of different risk factors lead to the development of deep vein thrombosis (DVT) or pulmonary embolism (PE). Surgery in general and orthopedic surgery in particular is however one of the most important single risk factors for DVT. Since these risk factors are cumulative [1] and many patients have multiple risk factors for DVT, the accumulated risk for VTE in orthopedic surgery can be

L.J. Lapidus, M.D., Ph.D.
Department of Clinical Science and Education,
Karolinska Institutet, Södersjukhuset Hospital, Stockholm,
Sjukhusbacken 10, 188 83 Stockholm, Sweden

Department of Orthopedics, Karolinska Institutet,
Södersjukhuset Hospital, Stockholm, Sjukhusbacken 10, 188 83 Stockholm, Sweden
e-mail: lasse.lapidus@sodersjukhuset.se

J.V. Llau (ed.), *Thromboembolism in Orthopedic Surgery*,
DOI 10.1007/978-1-4471-4336-9_3, © Springer-Verlag London 2013

Table 3.1 Risk factors for venous thromboembolism in orthopedics

Patient related	Age
	Previous venous thromboembolism
	Family history of venous thromboembolism
	Obesity
	Varicose veins
	Hormonal treatment
	Active cancer
Procedure related	Total hip arthroplasty
	Total knee arthroplasty
	Hip fracture and other lower limb fractures
	Plaster cast immobilization
	Multiple trauma
	Spinal cord injuries

very high for many patients (Table 3.1). After major orthopedic surgery, 40–80 % of the patients develop a thrombosis (mostly asymptomatic) in the absence of thromboprophylaxis [2], and in approximately 25 % of the patients, postoperative DVT also occurs in the contralateral leg [3, 4]. Although the relevance of asymptomatic DVT can be questioned, the high VTE incidence reflects the coagulopathy seen after surgery [5].

A detailed understanding of the pathophysiology of VTE was first published by a German pathologist, Rudolf Virchow (1821–1902), in the 1850s [6]. He presented the cornerstones for clot formation in the veins in the classic "Virchow's triad," which includes impaired blood flow (venous stasis), a change in the blood composition resulting in increased coagulability, and an injury of the blood vessel wall acting as a trigger factor for clot formation. Virchow postulated that all three factors need to be present for a thrombosis to develop. With this in mind, it is understandable that lower limb injuries and orthopedic surgery in the lower extremity is associated with an increased risk for developing DVT since all three components for clot formation usually are present. Local endothelial injuries to blood vessels are inevitable in surgery and often occur in trauma. Venous stasis is always present due to some grade of immobilization, and postoperative swelling and systemic coagulopathy occurs after major orthopedic surgery [3, 4]. Their mutual relation and importance for development of postoperative DVT is however unknown. The risk of postoperative VTEs remains increased for 2–3 months after major orthopedic surgery [7, 8] but the majority of thromboembolic events occur during the first postsurgical month [8].

The peak incidence of DVT seems to vary with the surgical procedure performed. After a total knee arthroplasty (TKA), 85 % of the DVTs diagnosed during the first postsurgical week were detected as early as the first day after surgery [9]. DVTs after total hip replacement (THR) seem to occur later, with a peak incidence 4 days after the surgery [10]. It is reasonable to believe that the extent of endothelial injury plays an important role for how fast the thrombosis actually develops. Possible mechanisms for late-occurring VTE have been related to prolonged activation of the coagulation system [5, 11]. A prolonged reduction in venous outflow has also been described, persisting for 6 weeks after THR [12, 13] but normalizing during the first week after TKA [14]. These findings suggest that there are some differences in the exact mechanism for how a DVT develops after surgery.

Risk Assessment

In the assessment of risk factors for specific procedures or injuries, it is important to remember the multifactorial etiology to VTE. In addition to the risk inherent to a specific clinical situation (e.g., specific injuries or specific surgical procedures), a variety of demographic characteristics may affect the risk for VTE. Also, other factors can alter the risk for VTE such as local traditions in the peroperative and postoperative setting, the type of anesthesia used during the surgery, time to ambulation after surgery, surgical technique, cemented or cementless prosthesis used in hip prosthesis surgery (which affects operating time, blood loss, etc.), modalities of physiotherapy, and the level of weight bearing after lower limb injuries. All these confounding factors may vary in time and place and possibly give unexpected results in clinical trials. For example, in the study by Sharrock et al. [15], the DVT incidence after TKA was evaluated. The only factor associated with a significant increased risk for DVT was one of the three surgeons. The authors found that this particular surgeon had his own method for deflating and reinflating the tourniquet without exsanguinating the limb after the cementing of the components was performed and concluded that this was the reason for the increased risk for DVT in this study.

Individual risk assessment may be of practical assistance in stratifying patients to different thromboprophylactic regimes according to the degree of risk for VTE. A number of simple risk assessment models have been developed which stratify patients into different risk categories. The ACCP group (American College of Chest Physicians) has simplified the risk assessment for surgical patients in a model involving four different VTE risk levels based on the type of surgery (e.g., minor or major), age (e.g., <40, 40–60, and >60 years), and the presence of additional risk factors (e.g., cancer or previous VTE) [16]. In the clinical situation, these models can provide a comprehensive guidance to the surgeon so that appropriate prophylaxis is provided to patients at risk for thrombosis. Furthermore, they allow physicians to follow a rational strategy with a systematic assessment of every patient in order to provide prophylaxis for similar patients in a reproducible fashion and in the long term, improve the clinical outcome. However, none of these risk assessment models has yet been consequently validated in a clinical setting where a risk assessment model is incorporated into the standard practical guidelines. In reality, there is an obvious risk for suboptimal compliance to a protocol with this type of individual approach to thromboprophylaxis since it is more complex to administer. The implementation of group-specific thromboprophylaxis protocols is possibly more efficient since they simplify the administration of thromboprophylaxis and might also increase the compliance with existing protocols.

VTE in Specific Orthopedic Procedures and Injuries

Elective Total Hip Replacement

Hip replacement surgery has become a model for VTE prevalence studies in the development of thromboprophylactic agents, and the high risk for VTE is well documented. Also, the pathophysiology of DVT after THR has been described, and the presence of the three cornerstones in Virchow's triad has been demonstrated in a number of studies.

- A peroperative local injury to the femoral vein is common and occurs during extensive flexion and rotation of the hip when preparing proximal femur for the femoral stem. The femoral vein is bent and compressed between femur and the pubic bone resulting in a local endothelial injury [13, 17–19]. It has also been demonstrated that the injury site can act as the primary clotting site for the DVTs [17, 18, 20–22]. As a consequence, the risk for proximal DVT is high after THR. There is no evidence suggesting that one surgical approach would be safer than others (i.e., the anterolateral approach or the posterolateral approach).
- A significant reduction of the venous outflow has been demonstrated. This venous stasis is persistent for weeks [12, 13] in contrast to knee prosthesis surgery where the venous outflow seems to normalize in 6 days after surgery [14].
- A systemic activation of the hemostatic system is known to occur, persisting for at least 4 weeks [5, 11].

Another factor to consider in THR is the use of spinal or epidural regional anesthesia, which is associated with a significant reduction in the incidence of postoperative DVT after THR, compared to general anesthesia, especially in the absence of other thromboprophylaxis [23]. However, this risk reduction is not strong enough to justify that pharmacological prophylaxis not being used (see below).

Total Knee Arthroplasty

The risk for VTE after TKA differs from that of THR in several aspects. With or without thromboprophylaxis, the total DVT rate is higher in TKA than in THR and the rate of distal DVT is higher in TKA than in THR [2]. The DVTs occur earlier in TKA compared to THR, and most DVTs after TKA occur during the first week with a peak incidence at 1 day after surgery [9]. Also, the pharmacological prophylaxis used has significantly lower efficacy in TKA than in THR. The use of tourniquet in TKA is one difference that might influence the clinical differences in the development of DVT in TKA compared with THR [15].

TKA performed in epidural anesthesia compared to general anesthesia reduced the risk for DVT (including proximal DVTs) in a study with 705 TKAs performed on 541 patients by a single surgeon. Preoperative and postoperative perfusion scans of the lungs and a venography of the operated limb were performed in all patients. The incidence of DVT was 48 and 64 % in the different groups in favor for patients operated in epidural anesthesia. The greatest reduction was in the occurrence of proximal DVT, which was identified in 9 % of the patients who had had general anesthesia but in only 4 % of those who had had epidural anesthesia ($p < 0.05$) [24].

Knee Arthroscopy

Arthroscopy and arthroscopy-assisted knee surgery (e.g., meniscectomy, synovectomy, and reconstruction of the cruciate ligaments) are some of the most common orthopedic procedures performed, and the risk for symptomatic VTE is very low. In a prospective study of 8,791 procedures, a symptomatic VTE incidence of less than 0.15 % was presented (with no fatal PE) [25]. In two other studies, with more than 9,850 procedures performed, the VTE incidence was 0.12 % with no fatal PEs [26, 27]. Other available studies permit a limited assessment of VTE risk factors among arthroscopy patients, but it appears that therapeutic arthroscopy is associated with a higher risk for VTE than diagnostic arthroscopy. Also, the tourniquet time appears to be a risk factor for VTE in knee arthroscopy, perhaps reflecting the complexity of the surgery performed. However, in other circumstances, the use of a tourniquet during lower limb surgery has also been shown to increase the risk for VTE [28].

The cumulative effect of multiple risk factors is illustrated in a prospective study [29] on 102 consecutive patients undergoing elective unilateral knee arthroscopy without thromboprophylaxis. Asymptomatic below-knee DVT in the operated leg occurred in eight patients (7.8 % of cases). The relative risk of DVT was higher (2.94, $p < 0.05$) among patients with two or more other relevant risk factors and among those with a history of thrombosis (8.2, $p < 0.005$).

Elective Spine Surgery

While the incidence of VTE after elective spine surgery appears to be considerably lower than that after major lower extremity surgery, some patients seem to be at higher risk for VTE. In a review article of 20 studies reporting complications after lumbar spinal fusions [30], the incidence of symptomatic DVT and PE was 3.7 and 2.2 %, respectively. In one of these studies [31], increased age and surgery of the lumbar spine (compared to the cervical spine) were independent predictors for DVT. Other possible risk factors include an anterior or combined anterior and posterior surgical approach, surgery for malignancy, a prolonged procedure, and reduced preoperative or postoperative mobility.

Multiple Trauma

Not only orthopedic surgery but also the trauma itself is an important risk factor for VTE. Independent risk factors for a VTE after trauma include spinal cord injury, pelvic fracture, and lower limb fracture [32, 33]. Preoperative DVTs occur frequently. Up to 35–60 % of patients with pelvic fractures have been found to have a DVT prior to surgery [34]. Preoperative DVTs are also common after femoral shaft fractures [35]. The significance of post-traumatic VTE was reported by Tuttle-Newhall et al. [36], who showed that PE increases the risk for a fatal outcome tenfold, from 2.6 to 26 %, after multiple trauma. Advanced age and lower extremity injury were identified as individual risk factors for VTE in this study. In another study on 716 multiple trauma patients, with injury severity score (ISS) of 9 or more, receiving no thromboprophylaxis, DVT screening was performed to evaluate the incidence of DVT and associated risk factors [33]. DVT was found in 201 of the 349 patients (58 %) with adequate venographic studies (only three with clinical symptoms), and proximal DVT was found in 63 patients (18 %). Additional three patients died of massive PE before venography could be performed. A multivariate regression analysis identified five independent risk factors for DVT:

- High age (OR 1.05 per year of age; 95 % CI: 1.03–1.06)
- Blood transfusion (OR 1.74; 95 % CI: 1.03–2.93)
- Surgery (OR 2.30; 95 % CI: 1.08–4.89)
- Fracture of the femur or tibia (OR 4.82; 95 % CI: 2.79–8.33)
- Spinal cord injury (OR 8.59; 95 % CI: 2.92–25.28)

Hip Fracture

It is well established that patients with hip fractures are at very high risk of VTE with DVT incidence rates of 50 and 27 % (total DVT and proximal DVT, respectively) without prophylaxis using screening contrast venography [37–42]. The rate of fatal PE is also significant, in the range of 1.4–7.5 % within 3 months. In an autopsy study performed between 1953 and 1992, fatal PE accounted for 14 % of all deaths after hip fracture surgery, being the fourth leading cause of death in this group of patients [43]. In addition to the initial injury and its surgical repair, factors that may further increase the risk of VTE after hip fracture surgery include advanced age and delayed surgery [43–46], while the influence of the type of anesthesia (general anesthesia or regional anesthesia) remains uncertain [47], possibly with marginal advantages for regional anesthesia compared to general anesthesia in patients with femoral neck fracture [48].

In patients with hip fractures, there is sometimes a delay to hospital admission affecting the risk for VTE. In one study, patients admitted more than 2 days after the injury causing the fracture had a significantly increased risk for DVT (55 %, 6 out of 11) compared to patients admitted within 2 days of the injury (6 %, 7 out of 122) [45].

Even if the total number of patients admitted late was low ($n = 11$), it is worthwhile mentioning that out of 13 patients with DVT, 6 patients had ipsilateral DVT, 3 patients had contralateral DVT and 4 patients had bilateral DVT. These results highlight the obvious risk of fatal VTE events in patients with a hip fracture.

More frequently, there is a delay between hospital admission and surgery, while the patient is being assessed and waiting for operating room availability. As a consequence, a DVT may develop between the time of injury and the fixation of the fracture, contributing to the high DVT incidence in hip fracture patients [43, 45, 46, 49, 50]. In one hip fracture study where surgery was delayed by at least 48 h, 21 patients were screened with venography before surgery. DVT occurred in 62 % of patients, and proximal DVT occurred in 14 % [46]. Also, these results highlight the potential risk for fatal VTE events, and therefore, if surgery is likely to be delayed, strong consideration should be given to commencing prophylaxis during the preoperative period in patients admitted due to a hip fracture.

Long Bone Fracture Distal to the Hip

The risk for DVT in long bone fractures distal to the hip was evaluated in a study by Abelseth et al. [35]. The incidence of VTE in 102 patients with lower limb fractures was evaluated by venography approximately 9 days after surgery. The DVT incidence after a femoral shaft fracture, a proximal tibia fracture, a tibial shaft fracture, and a distal tibia fracture was 40, 43, 22 and 12 %, respectively. Four patients had symptoms indicating a PE, but only in one case was the PE confirmed. All patients were operated on and mobilized without the use of a plaster cast. Proximal fractures were associated with a higher risk of DVT compared to more distal fractures.

Plaster Cast Immobilization of Lower Limb Injury

The increased risk for VTE after plaster cast immobilization of lower limb fractures is particularly well documented, reported as early as 1944 [51]. Later, in a prospective observational study conducted in 1968 by Hjelmstedt [52], the natural history of VTE was evaluated in 79 patients treated for a tibial fracture. The overall DVT incidence was 45 % (proximal DVT in 8 % of patients), and a fatal PE was found at autopsy in one patient. Only one third of the DVTs were symptomatic. Surgical treatment of the fracture seemed to be an additional risk factor with a DVT incidence of 71 % for surgically treated patients and 39 % for patients treated nonoperatively. More recent studies assessing the efficacy of thromboprophylaxis during plaster cast immobilization after lower limb injuries confirm a high risk for DVT in patients with fracture as well as soft tissue injuries [53–57], regardless if the patients are treated surgically or not. Due to the high number of asymptomatic DVTs in these studies as well as uncertainty regarding the efficacy and unclear cost-benefit outcome for thromboprophylaxis, still, no general consensus exists for thromboprophylaxis during lower limb plaster cast immobilization [2].

Other studies assessing specific risk factors in plaster cast immobilization have not been found, but it is possible that non-weight bearing compared to fully weight bearing in plaster may increase the risk for DVT. Other clinical situations that is related to a suspected increased risk for DVT in plaster cast immobilization (and when prophylaxis is recommended) include high age, history of VTE, pregnancy and hormone replacement therapy, the latter especially in combination with smoking.

Foot Surgery

Surgical procedures in the foot seem to have limited risk for VTE without thromboprophylaxis; symptomatic DVT incidence less than 0.5 % has been reported in large materials [58, 59]. The use of plaster cast immobilization could possibly increase this risk.

Upper Extremity Surgery

VTE following upper extremity surgery is rare. One retrospective study reviewed 2,885 consecutive primary shoulder arthroplasties performed in a single institution over 20 years [60]. Five patients sustained nonfatal postoperative PE; the authors concluded that PE is an uncommon complication after shoulder arthroplasty, but surgeons should have a high degree of suspicion if patients have respiratory problems after surgery.

Spinal Cord Injury

Patients with paralytic spinal cord injury represent another dignity with regards to the risk for VTE which is among the highest among all hospital admissions [61]. The overall incidence of DVT and PE within 3 months is 38 % and approximately 5 %, respectively [62]. The risk appears to be greatest during the first 2 weeks after injury, and fatal PE is rare >3 months after injury [62–64].

The cause of the decrease in clinically evident PE after 3 months is unknown. However, a number of changes associated with chronic paralysis may be involved, including a gradual atrophy of the leg muscles and, in many individuals, the development of small caliber collateral veins around organized old venous thrombi obstructing the major deep leg veins [65].

Other Clinical Situations of Consideration

Type of Anesthesia

The use of regional anesthesia (spinal or epidural) is associated with a significant reduction in the incidence of postoperative DVT (especially proximal DVT) after THR and TKA compared to general anesthesia. This has been evaluated in a few randomized studies [66–71] and in a review article [23]. In the absence of pharmacological thromboprophylaxis, a relative risk reduction of 46–55 % was identified in patients with regional anesthesia, but together with pharmacological prophylaxis, the DVT incidence was equalized between the groups. However, regional anesthesia alone cannot be considered adequate thromboprophylaxis because the risk of VTE remains unacceptably high without pharmacological thromboprophylaxis. Several confounding risk factors compromise the interpretation of studies on this topic.

The Use of a Pneumatic Tourniquet in the Lower Limb

Present studies give no conclusive data on the role of lower limb pneumatic tourniquet and the development of thrombosis, but in a recent meta-analysis, the risk for VTE with or without the use of tourniquet in TKA surgery was evaluated [72]. In the pooled results including 634 TKAs, there was a significant increased risk for clinical thromboembolic events when a tourniquet was used during surgery. Symptomatic thromboembolic events occurred in 13.0 and 6.1 % of patients in the tourniquet and non-tourniquet group, respectively (RR 1.91, CI; 1.05–3.49). In the subgroup analysis, there was a trend to increased risk for both symptomatic DVT (14 % vs. 7.1 %) and PE (9.8 % vs. 3.4 %) in the tourniquet group compared to the non-tourniquet group.

Some factors that might promote the development of endothelial injury and thrombosis when using a lower limb tourniquet are if the limb is exsanguinated or not before the cuff is inflated, the duration of tourniquet applied, the type of cuff used, and the cuff pressure used during surgery. The use of tourniquet in surgery has been shown to induce local thrombogenic and fibrinolytic activity, but this activity itself is not sufficient to activate systemic markers of thrombin generation and fibrinolysis [73–76]. The critical point seems to be the deflation of the tourniquet when the surgical procedure has been performed, even fatal PEs have been reported [77, 78].

Immobility

Inadequate mobilization such as bed rest predisposes for VTE. In one study, 15 % of patients on bed rest for less than 1 week before death had a DVT at autopsy, while the DVT incidence increased to 80 % in patients in bed for more than 1 week [79].

It is possible that elderly people, who are well mobilized during hospitalization, become more or less bedridden at home after discharge and are therefore at increased risk for late VTE.

Malignancy

It is reasonable to believe that the substantial risk for VTE following orthopedic surgery in normal conditions is likely to be even higher for patients with an ongoing malignancy. Due to confounding factors, it is however difficult to estimate the additional increase in VTE risk for the malignancy per se. Different cancers also have different thrombogenic properties; advanced cancers (breast, lung, brain, pelvis, rectum, pancreas, and gastrointestinal tract) are associated with a high incidence of VTE, and ongoing treatment with chemotherapy increases the risk further, two- to three-fold increased risk has been reported [80–82]. Besides the additional thrombotic stimulus from the malignant disease, it is possible that the recovery period is prolonged and the grade of immobilization is increased.

Pregnancy/Puerperium

The increased risk for VTE during pregnancy and the postpartum period needs special attention to minimize the risk for VTE in case of orthopedic injuries or orthopedic surgery. Thromboprophylaxis should be considered even after minor procedures or plaster cast immobilization of the lower extremity.

Oral Contraceptives

In case of significant orthopedic injuries or orthopedic surgery, it is mandatory to rule out additional risk factors for VTE, such us ongoing medication with oral contraceptives and possibly hormone replacement therapy. Even if no randomized studies have been performed, it is reasonable to consider prolonged thromboprophylaxis and if appropriate, discontinue the medication in case of elective surgery. The increased risk for VTE was evaluated in a recent case-control study by Lidegaard [83] who found an incidence of VTE in young women between 1 and 3 per 10,000 per year. Pregnancy increases this risk 5 times, low-dose third-generation oral contraceptives 4 times and low-dose second-generation oral contraceptives 3 times. In women receiving hormone replacement therapy (HRT), the estrogen dose is generally 20–25 % of that contained in modern oral contraceptives [84]. Despite the much lower biological potency, women taking HRT have a two- to four-fold increased risk of idiopathic venous thrombosis compared with women not taking

HRT [85–88]. Like women receiving estrogens for contraception or menopause, men receiving estrogen therapy for prostate cancer are also at increased risk for VTE [89].

References

1. Deehan DJ, Siddique M, Weir DJ, Pinder IM, Lingard EM. Postphlebitic syndrome after total knee arthroplasty: 405 patients examined 2–10 years after surgery. Acta Orthop Scand. 2001;72(1):42–5.
2. Geerts WH, Pineo GF, Heit JA, Bergqvist D, Lassen MR, Colwell CW, et al. Prevention of venous thromboembolism: the seventh ACCP conference on antithrombotic and thrombolytic therapy. Chest. 2004;126(3 Suppl):338S–400. doi:10.1378/chest.126.3_suppl.338S.
3. Cruickshank MK, Levine MN, Hirsh J, Turpie AG, Powers P, Jay R, et al. An evaluation of impedance plethysmography and 125I-fibrinogen leg scanning in patients following hip surgery. Thromb Haemost. 1989;62(3):830–4.
4. Comp PC, Spiro TE, Friedman RJ, Whitsett TL, Johnson GJ, Gardiner Jr GA, et al. Prolonged enoxaparin therapy to prevent venous thromboembolism after primary hip or knee replacement. Enoxaparin Clinical Trial Group. J Bone Joint Surg Am. 2001;83-A(3):336–45.
5. Andersen BS. Postoperative activation of the haemostatic system – influence of prolonged thromboprophylaxis in patients undergoing total hip arthroplasty. Haemostasis. 1997;27(5):219–27.
6. Virchow R. Abhandlungen zur Wissenschaftligen Medicin. Frankfurt: Von Medinger Sohn&Co; 1856.
7. White RH, Romano PS, Zhou H, Rodrigo J, Bargar W. Incidence and time course of thromboembolic outcomes following total hip or knee arthroplasty. Arch Intern Med. 1998;158(14): 1525–31.
8. Bjornara BT, Gudmundsen TE, Dahl OE. Frequency and timing of clinical venous thromboembolism after major joint surgery. J Bone Joint Surg Br. 2006;88(3):386–91.
9. Maynard MJ, Sculco TP, Ghelman B. Progression and regression of deep vein thrombosis after total knee arthroplasty. Clin Orthop Relat Res. 1991;273:125–30.
10. Sikorski JM, Hampson WG, Staddon GE. The natural history and aetiology of deep vein thrombosis after total hip replacement. J Bone Joint Surg Br. 1981;63-B(2):171–7.
11. Dahl OE, Pedersen T, Kierulf P, Westvik AB, Lund P, Arnesen H, et al. Sequential intrapulmonary and systemic activation of coagulation and fibrinolysis during and after total hip replacement surgery. Thromb Res. 1993;70(6):451–8.
12. McNally MA, Mollan RA. Total hip replacement, lower limb blood flow and venous thrombogenesis. J Bone Joint Surg Br. 1993;75(4):640–4.
13. Warwick D, Martin AG, Glew D, Bannister GC. Measurement of femoral vein blood flow during total hip replacement. Duplex ultrasound imaging with and without the use of a foot pump. J Bone Joint Surg Br. 1994;76(6):918–21.
14. McNally MA, Bahadur R, Cooke EA, Mollan RA. Venous haemodynamics in both legs after total knee replacement. J Bone Joint Surg Br. 1997;79(4):633–7.
15. Sharrock NE, Hargett MJ, Urquhart B, Peterson MG, Ranawat C, Insall J, et al. Factors affecting deep vein thrombosis rate following total knee arthroplasty under epidural anesthesia. J Arthroplasty. 1993;8(2):133–9.
16. Geerts WH, Heit JA, Clagett GP, Pineo GF, Colwell CW, Anderson Jr FA, et al. Prevention of venous thromboembolism. Chest. 2001;119(1 Suppl):132S–75.
17. Stamatakis JD, Kakkar VV, Sagar S, Lawrence D, Nairn D, Bentley PG. Femoral vein thrombosis and total hip replacement. Br Med J. 1977;2(6081):223–5.
18. Planes A, Vochelle N, Fagola M. Total hip replacement and deep vein thrombosis. A venographic and necropsy study. J Bone Joint Surg Br. 1990;72(1):9–13.

19. Binns M, Pho R. Femoral vein occlusion during hip arthroplasty. Clin Orthop Relat Res. 1990;255:168–72.
20. Nillius AS, Nylander G. Deep vein thrombosis after total hip replacement: a clinical and phlebographic study. Br J Surg. 1979;66(5):324–6.
21. Kalebo P, Anthmyr BA, Eriksson BI, Zachrisson BE. Phlebographic findings in venous thrombosis following total hip replacement. Acta Radiol. 1990;31(3):259–63.
22. Ascani A, Radicchia S, Parise P, Nenci GG, Agnelli G. Distribution and occlusiveness of thrombi in patients with surveillance detected deep vein thrombosis after hip surgery. Thromb Haemost. 1996;75(2):239–41.
23. Prins MH, Hirsh J. A comparison of general anesthesia and regional anesthesia as a risk factor for deep vein thrombosis following hip surgery: a critical review. Thromb Haemost. 1990;64(4): 497–500.
24. Sharrock NE, Haas SB, Hargett MJ, Urquhart B, Insall JN, Scuderi G. Effects of epidural anesthesia on the incidence of deep-vein thrombosis after total knee arthroplasty. J Bone Joint Surg Am. 1991;73(4):502–6.
25. Small NC. Complications in arthroscopic surgery performed by experienced arthroscopists. Arthroscopy. 1988;4(3):215–21.
26. Bamford DJ, Paul AS, Noble J, Davies DR. Avoidable complications of arthroscopic surgery. J R Coll Surg Edinb. 1993;38(2):92–5.
27. Dahl OE, Gudmundsen TE, Haukeland L. Late occurring clinical deep vein thrombosis in joint-operated patients. Acta Orthop Scand. 2000;71(1):47–50.
28. Warwick DJ, Whitehouse S. Symptomatic venous thromboembolism after total knee replacement. J Bone Joint Surg Br. 1997;79(5):780–6.
29. Delis KT, Hunt N, Strachan RK, Nicolaides AN. Incidence, natural history and risk factors of deep vein thrombosis in elective knee arthroscopy. Thromb Haemost. 2001;86(3): 817–21.
30. Turner JA, Ersek M, Herron L, Haselkorn J, Kent D, Ciol MA, et al. Patient outcomes after lumbar spinal fusions. JAMA. 1992;268(7):907–11.
31. Oda T, Fuji T, Kato Y, Fujita S, Kanemitsu N. Deep venous thrombosis after posterior spinal surgery. Spine (Phila Pa 1976). 2000;25(22):2962–7.
32. Meissner MH, Chandler WL, Elliott JS. Venous thromboembolism in trauma: a local manifestation of systemic hypercoagulability? J Trauma. 2003;54(2):224–31.
33. Geerts WH, Code KI, Jay RM, Chen E, Szalai JP. A prospective study of venous thromboembolism after major trauma. N Engl J Med. 1994;331(24):1601–6.
34. Montgomery KD, Geerts WH, Potter HG, Helfet DL. Thromboembolic complications in patients with pelvic trauma. Clin Orthop Relat Res. 1996;329:68–87.
35. Abelseth G, Buckley RE, Pineo GE, Hull R, Rose MS. Incidence of deep-vein thrombosis in patients with fractures of the lower extremity distal to the hip. J Orthop Trauma. 1996;10(4): 230–5.
36. Tuttle-Newhall JE, Rutledge R, Hultman CS, Fakhry SM. Statewide, population-based, time-series analysis of the frequency and outcome of pulmonary embolus in 318,554 trauma patients. J Trauma. 1997;42(1):90–9.
37. Powers PJ, Gent M, Jay RM, Julian DH, Turpie AG, Levine M, et al. A randomized trial of less intense postoperative warfarin or aspirin therapy in the prevention of venous thromboembolism after surgery for fractured hip. Arch Intern Med. 1989;149(4):771–4.
38. Snook GA, Chrisman OD, Wilson TC. Thromboembolism after surgical treatment of hip fractures. Clin Orthop Relat Res. 1981;(155):21–4.
39. Agnelli G, Cosmi B, Di Filippo P, Ranucci V, Veschi F, Longetti M, et al. A randomised, double-blind, placebo-controlled trial of dermatan sulphate for prevention of deep vein thrombosis in hip fracture. Thromb Haemost. 1992;67(2):203–8.
40. Hamilton HW, Crawford JS, Gardiner JH, Wiley AM. Venous thrombosis in patients with fracture of the upper end of the femur. A phlebographic study of the effect of prophylactic anticoagulation. J Bone Joint Surg Br. 1970;52(2):268–89.

41. Lowe GD, Campbell AF, Meek DR, Forbes CD, Prentice CR. Subcutaneous ancrod in prevention of deep-vein thrombosis after operation for fractured neck of femur. Lancet. 1978;2(8092 Pt 1):698–700.
42. Rogers PH, Walsh PN, Marder VJ, Bosak GC, Lachman JW, Ritchie WG, et al. Controlled trial of low-dose heparin and sulfinpyrazone to prevent venous thromboembolism after operation on the hip. J Bone Joint Surg Am. 1978;60(6):758–62.
43. Perez JV, Warwick DJ, Case CP, Bannister GC. Death after proximal femoral fracture – an autopsy study. Injury. 1995;26(4):237–40.
44. Schroder HM, Andreassen M. Autopsy-verified major pulmonary embolism after hip fracture. Clin Orthop Relat Res. 1993;293:196–203.
45. Hefley Jr FG, Nelson CL, Puskarich-May CL. Effect of delayed admission to the hospital on the preoperative prevalence of deep-vein thrombosis associated with fractures about the hip. J Bone Joint Surg Am. 1996;78(4):581–3.
46. Zahn HR, Skinner JA, Porteous MJ. The preoperative prevalence of deep vein thrombosis in patients with femoral neck fractures and delayed operation. Injury. 1999;30(9):605–7.
47. Sorenson RM, Pace NL. Anesthetic techniques during surgical repair of femoral neck fractures. A meta-analysis. Anesthesiology. 1992;77(6):1095–104.
48. Urwin SC, Parker MJ, Griffiths R. General versus regional anaesthesia for hip fracture surgery: a meta-analysis of randomized trials. Br J Anaesth. 2000;84(4):450–5.
49. Roberts TS, Nelson CL, Barnes CL, Ferris EJ, Holder JC, Boone DW. The preoperative prevalence and postoperative incidence of thromboembolism in patients with hip fractures treated with dextran prophylaxis. Clin Orthop Relat Res. 1990;255:198–203.
50. Girasole GJ, Cuomo F, Denton JR, O'Connor D, Ernst A. Diagnosis of deep vein thrombosis in elderly hip-fracture patients by using the duplex scanning technique. Orthop Rev. 1994;23(5):411–6.
51. Bauer G. Thrombosis following leg injuries. Acta Chir Scand. 1944;90:229–49.
52. Hjelmstedt A. Incidence of thrombosis in patients with tibial fractures. Acta Chir Scand. 1968;134(3):209–18.
53. Kujath P, Spannagel U, Habscheid W. Incidence and prophylaxis of deep venous thrombosis in outpatients with injury of the lower limb. Haemostasis. 1993;23 Suppl 1:20–6.
54. Jorgensen PS, Warming T, Hansen K, Paltved C, Vibeke Berg H, Jensen R, et al. Low molecular weight heparin (Innohep) as thromboprophylaxis in outpatients with a plaster cast: a venografic controlled study. Thromb Res. 2002;105(6):477–80.
55. Lassen MR, Borris LC, Nakov RL. Use of the low-molecular-weight heparin reviparin to prevent deep-vein thrombosis after leg injury requiring immobilization. N Engl J Med. 2002;347(10):726–30.
56. Lapidus LJ, Rosfors S, Ponzer S, Levander C, Elvin A, Larfars G, et al. Prolonged thromboprophylaxis with dalteparin after surgical treatment of achilles tendon rupture: a randomized, placebo-controlled study. J Orthop Trauma. 2007;21(1):52–7.
57. Lapidus LJ, Ponzer S, Elvin A, Levander C, Larfars G, Rosfors S, et al. Prolonged thromboprophylaxis with Dalteparin during immobilization after ankle fracture surgery: a randomized placebo-controlled, double-blind study. Acta Orthop. 2007;78(4):528–35.
58. Mizel MS, Temple HT, Michelson JD, Alvarez RG, Clanton TO, Frey CC, et al. Thromboembolism after foot and ankle surgery. A multicenter study. Clin Orthop Relat Res. 1998;348:180–5.
59. Wukich DK, Waters DH. Thromboembolism following foot and ankle surgery: a case series and literature review. J Foot Ankle Surg. 2008;47(3):243–9.
60. Sperling JW, Cofield RH. Pulmonary embolism following shoulder arthroplasty. J Bone Joint Surg Am. 2002;84-A(11):1939–41.
61. Consortium for Spinal Cord Medicine. Prevention of thromboembolism in spinal cord injury. J Spinal Cord Med. 1997;20:259–83.
62. Waring WP, Karunas RS. Acute spinal cord injuries and the incidence of clinically occurring thromboembolic disease. Paraplegia. 1991;29(1):8–16.

63. Green D, Lee MY, Lim AC, Chmiel JS, Vetter M, Pang T, et al. Prevention of thromboembolism after spinal cord injury using low-molecular-weight heparin. Ann Intern Med. 1990;113(8):571–4.
64. Green D, Lee MY, Ito VY, Cohn T, Press J, Filbrandt PR, et al. Fixed- vs adjusted-dose heparin in the prophylaxis of thromboembolism in spinal cord injury. JAMA. 1988;260(9):1255–8.
65. Anderson Jr FA, Spencer FA. Risk factors for venous thromboembolism. Circulation. 2003;107(23 Suppl 1):I9–16.
66. Davis FM, Laurenson VG, Gillespie WJ, Foate J, Seagar AD. Leg blood flow during total hip replacement under spinal or general anaesthesia. Anaesth Intensive Care. 1989;17(2):136–43.
67. Modig J, Hjelmstedt A, Sahlstedt B, Maripuu E. Comparative influences of epidural and general anaesthesia on deep venous thrombosis and pulmonary embolism after total hip replacement. Acta Chir Scand. 1981;147(2):125–30.
68. Modig J, Borg T, Karlstrom G, Maripuu E, Sahlstedt B. Thromboembolism after total hip replacement: role of epidural and general anesthesia. Anesth Analg. 1983;62(2):174–80.
69. Modig J. The role of lumbar epidural anaesthesia as antithrombotic prophylaxis in total hip replacement. Acta Chir Scand. 1985;151(7):589–94.
70. Nielsen PT, Jorgensen LN, Albrecht-Beste E, Leffers AM, Rasmussen LS. Lower thrombosis risk with epidural blockade in knee arthroplasty. Acta Orthop Scand. 1990;61(1):29–31.
71. Thorburn J, Louden JR, Vallance R. Spinal and general anaesthesia in total hip replacement: frequency of deep vein thrombosis. Br J Anaesth. 1980;52(11):1117–21.
72. Tai TW, Lin CJ, Jou IM, Chang CW, Lai KA, Yang CY. Tourniquet use in total knee arthroplasty: a meta-analysis. Knee Surg Sports Traumatol Arthrosc. 2011;19(7):1121–30.
73. Reikeras O, Clementsen T. Time course of thrombosis and fibrinolysis in total knee arthroplasty with tourniquet application. Local versus systemic activations. J Thromb Thrombolysis. 2009;28(4):425–8.
74. Petaja J, Myllynen P, Myllyla G, Vahtera E. Fibrinolysis after application of a pneumatic tourniquet. Acta Chir Scand. 1987;153(11–12):647–51.
75. Klenerman L, Chakrabarti R, Mackie I, Brozovic M, Stirling Y. Changes in haemostatic system after application of a tourniquet. Lancet. 1977;1(8019):970–2.
76. Sharrock NE, Go G, Williams-Russo P, Haas SB, Harpel PC. Comparison of extradural and general anaesthesia on the fibrinolytic response to total knee arthroplasty. Br J Anaesth. 1997;79(1):29–34.
77. Pollard BJ, Lovelock HA, Jones RM. Fatal pulmonary embolism secondary to limb exsanguination. Anesthesiology. 1983;58(4):373–4.
78. McGrath BJ, Hsia J, Epstein B. Massive pulmonary embolism following tourniquet deflation. Anesthesiology. 1991;74(3):618–20.
79. Gibbs NM. Venous thrombosis of the lower limbs with particular reference to bed-rest. Br J Surg. 1957;45(191):209–36.
80. Rahr HB, Sorensen JV. Venous thromboembolism and cancer. Blood Coagul Fibrinolysis. 1992;3(4):451–60.
81. Clahsen PC, van de Velde CJ, Julien JP, Floiras JL, Mignolet FY. Thromboembolic complications after perioperative chemotherapy in women with early breast cancer: a European Organization for Research and Treatment of Cancer Breast Cancer Cooperative Group study. J Clin Oncol. 1994;12(6):1266–71.
82. Lieberman JS, Borrero J, Urdaneta E, Wright IS. Thrombophlebitis and cancer. JAMA. 1961;177:542–5.
83. Lidegaard O, Edstrom B, Kreiner S. Oral contraceptives and venous thromboembolism: a five-year national case-control study. Contraception. 2002;65(3):187–96.
84. Grady D, Applegate W, Bush T, Furberg C, Riggs B, Hulley SB. Heart and Estrogen/progestin Replacement Study (HERS): design, methods, and baseline characteristics. Control Clin Trials. 1998;19(4):314–35.

85. Grodstein F, Stampfer MJ, Goldhaber SZ, Manson JE, Colditz GA, Speizer FE, et al. Prospective study of exogenous hormones and risk of pulmonary embolism in women. Lancet. 1996;348(9033):983–7.
86. Daly E, Vessey MP, Hawkins MM, Carson JL, Gough P, Marsh S. Risk of venous thromboembolism in users of hormone replacement therapy. Lancet. 1996;348(9033):977–80.
87. Lowe G, Woodward M, Vessey M, Rumley A, Gough P, Daly E. Thrombotic variables and risk of idiopathic venous thromboembolism in women aged 45–64 years. Relationships to hormone replacement therapy. Thromb Haemost. 2000;83(4):530–5.
88. Varas-Lorenzo C, Garcia-Rodriguez LA, Cattaruzzi C, Troncon MG, Agostinis L, Perez-Gutthann S. Hormone replacement therapy and the risk of hospitalization for venous thromboembolism: a population-based study in southern Europe. Am J Epidemiol. 1998;147(4): 387–90.
89. Lundgren R, Sundin T, Colleen S, Lindstedt E, Wadstrom L, Carlsson S, et al. Cardiovascular complications of estrogen therapy for nondisseminated prostatic carcinoma. A preliminary report from a randomized multicenter study. Scand J Urol Nephrol. 1986;20(2):101–5.

Chapter 4
Diagnosis and Treatment of Deep Vein Thrombosis and Pulmonary Embolism After Major Joint Surgery

Manuel Monreal and Juan I. Arcelus

Abstract Pulmonary embolism (PE) and deep vein thrombosis (DVT) are two clinical presentations of venous thromboembolism (VTE) and share the same predisposing factors. In a study by our group, the Spanish National Discharge Database was used to assess the frequency and clinical impact of venous VTE after elective total knee (TKA) or hip (THA) arthroplasty. In all, 58,037 patients underwent TKA, and 31,769 underwent THA. Of these, 179 (0.20 %) were diagnosed with symptomatic PE, 470 (0.52 %) were diagnosed with DVT, and 106 (0.12 %) died during the first 3 months after surgery. Mean hospital stay was significantly longer in patients who developed VTE than in those who did not. Of 106 patients who died, 20 (19 %) had been diagnosed with PE.

The first step in diagnosis VTE is the suspicion. Acute VTE should be suspected in patients with a combination of suggestive symptoms and/or signs. Most patients with confirmed PE do not have clinically evident DVT, and around 30 % of patients with symptomatic DVT have asymptomatic PE. The objectives of VTE treatment are to improve acute symptoms and to prevent thrombus extension, early recurrence, and death from PE. In most patients, the initial treatment of DVT and PE is similar since both conditions are considered different manifestations of the same disease. Anticoagulation remains the mainstay of VTE treatment.

Keywords Deep vein thrombosis • Pulmonary embolism • Knee arthroplasty • Hip arthroplasty • Diagnosis • Treatment

M. Monreal, M.D., Ph.D. (✉)
Department of Internal Medicine, Hospital Germans Trias I Pujol,
Badalona, Barcelona 08916, Spain
e-mail: mmonreal.germanstrias@gencat.cat

J.I. Arcelus, M.D., Ph.D.
Department of Surgery, Hospital Universitario Virgen de las Nieves,
University of Granada, Calle Madrid s/n, Granada 18071, Spain
e-mail: j.arcelus@telefonica.net

J.V. Llau (ed.), *Thromboembolism in Orthopedic Surgery*,
DOI 10.1007/978-1-4471-4336-9_4, © Springer-Verlag London 2013

Pulmonary embolism (PE) and deep vein thrombosis (DVT) are two clinical presentations of venous thromboembolism (VTE) and share the same predisposing factors. In most cases, PE is a consequence of DVT. Among patients with proximal DVT, about 50 % have an associated, often clinically asymptomatic, PE at lung scan.

In this chapter, we will review the diagnosis and treatment key points. We will develop the concept that diagnosis of VTE is commonly based in the suspicion as first step, supported by the results of the algorithms, and confirmed by the imaging test (venous ultrasound in DVT and computed tomography pulmonary angiography in PE). In reference to the treatment, the anticoagulant therapy is the cornerstone for the management of VTE, although if the patient has a PE with hemodynamic instability, the thrombolytic therapy should be in consideration.

Diagnosis

Venous Thromboembolism in the Spanish National Discharge Database (SNDD)

In a study by our group, the SNDD during the years 2005–2006 was used to assess the frequency and clinical impact of venous VTE after elective total knee (TKA) or hip (THA) arthroplasty [1]. In all, 58,037 patients underwent TKA, and 31,769 underwent THA. Their clinical characteristics are depicted in Table 4.1. There were 31,327 men (35 %) and 58,479 women, their mean age was 71 years, and the frequency of underlying diseases was as follows: hypertension 37 %, diabetes 11 %, chronic lung disease 5.2 %, obesity 4.8 %, ischemic heart disease 3.2 %, chronic heart failure 1.6 %, and cancer 1.0 %.

Of 58,037 patients undergoing TKA, 106 (0.18 %) were diagnosed with symptomatic PE, 330 (0.57 %) were diagnosed with DVT, and 54 (0.09 %) died during the first 3 months after surgery. Mean hospital stay was significantly longer in patients who developed VTE than in those who did not (14 ± 11 vs. 9.1 ± 5.8 days; $p < 0.001$). Most DVT events (77 %) and half of the PEs (53 %) were detected during hospital stay. Of 54 patients who died, 13 (24 %) had been diagnosed with PE and 2 (3.70 %) with DVT.

Of 31,769 patients undergoing elective THA, 73 (0.23 %) were diagnosed with symptomatic PE, 140 (0.44 %) with DVT, and 52 (0.16 %) died during the 3-month study period. Mean hospital stay was again significantly longer in those who developed VTE than in those who did not (19 ± 18 vs. 10 ± 6.7 days; $p < 0.001$). Most DVT events (67 %) and 42 % of the PEs were detected during hospital stay. Of 52 patients who died, 7 (13.5 %) had been diagnosed with PE.

Table 4.1 Univariable analysis for VTE for 58,037 patients undergoing TKA and 31,769 undergoing THA in the Spanish National Discharge Database

	VTE after TKA	No VTE after TKA	VTE after THA	No VTE after THA
Patients, *N*	436	57,601	213	31,556
Clinical characteristics				
Age (mean years ± SD)	71 ± 6.7	71 ± 7.3	69 ± 10	67 ± 12
Gender (males)	89 (20 %)**	15,330 (27 %)	113 (53 %)	15,795 (50 %)
Hospital stay (mean days ± SD)	14 ± 11***	9.1 ± 5.8	19 ± 18***	10 ± 6.7
Hospital stay > 10 days	243 (56 %)***	14,265 (25 %)	130 (61 %)***	9,439 (30 %)
Underlying diseases				
Obesity	42 (9.6 %)***	3,276 (5.7 %)	10 (4.7 %)	1,004 (3.2 %)
Chronic lung disease	31 (7.1 %)*	2,852 (5.0 %)	21 (9.9 %)**	1,758 (5.6 %)
Chronic heart failure	11 (2.5 %)	941 (1.6 %)	3 (1.4 %)	444 (1.4 %)
Diabetes	51 (12 %)	6,918 (12 %)	9 (4.2 %)*	2,662 (8.4 %)
Arterial hypertension	200 (46 %)*	23,525 (41 %)	71 (33 %)	9,666 (31 %)
Ischemic heart disease	20 (4.6 %)	1,816 (3.2 %)	10 (4.7 %)	1,028 (3.3 %)
Cancer	7 (1.6 %)*	444 (0.8 %)	5 (2.3 %)	423 (1.3 %)
Venous thromboembolism				
DVT during hospital stay	254 (58 %)	–	94 (44 %)	–
PE during hospital stay	56 (13 %)	–	31 (16 %)	–
DVT after discharge	76 (17 %)	–	46 (22 %)	–
PE after discharge	50 (11 %)	–	42 (20 %)	–
Any VTE	436 (100 %)	–	213 (100 %)	–

VTE venous thromboembolism, *TKA* total knee arthroplasty, *THA* total hip arthroplasty, *SD* standard deviation, *DVT* deep vein thrombosis, *PE* pulmonary embolism

Comparisons between patients with or without the event: *$p < 0.05$; **$p < 0.01$; ***$p < 0.001$

Clinical Presentation of VTE in Patients Undergoing Major Hip Surgery in the RIETE Registry

The "Registro Informatizado de Enfermedad TromboEmbólica" (RIETE) initiative is an ongoing, international (Spain, France, Italy, Israel, Germany, Republic of Macedonia, Switzerland, Brazil, Argentina), multicenter, and prospective registry of consecutive patients presenting with symptomatic acute VTE confirmed by objective tests [2–4]. We evaluated the clinical characteristics, time course, and diagnostic tests of 889 patients who developed symptomatic, acute pulmonary embolism (PE) or deep vein thrombosis (DVT) after major joint surgery (TKA, THA, or hip fracture) [5].

Overall, 457 (51 %) patients had clinically overt PE, and 432 (49 %) had only DVT, as shown in Table 4.2. The most common symptom in patients presenting with acute PE was dyspnea (87 %). Only 46 % of PE patients experienced chest pain, 16 % presented with syncope, and 3.7 % had hemoptysis. One in every four

Table 4.2 Clinical characteristics of patients with pulmonary embolism in the RIETE registry

	TKA	THA	Hip fracture	p value
Patients, *N*	166	152	157	
Initial VTE presentation				
Chest pain	79 (48 %)	67 (45 %)	62 (41 %)	0.416
Dyspnea	137 (84 %)	121 (81 %)	141 (91 %)	0.042
Hemoptysis	4 (2.5 %)	7 (4.7 %)	6 (4.0 %)	0.552
Syncope	24 (15 %)	29 (20 %)	19 (13 %)	0.237
SBP < 100 mmHg	21 (13 %)	21 (14 %)	18 (12 %)	0.824
Sat O_2 < 90 %	26 (23 %)	35 (32 %)	47 (44 %)	0.003
Heart rate > 110 bpm	24 (18 %)	27 (22 %)	33 (28 %)	0.151
Time from surgery to PE (days)	18 ± 18	27 ± 20	22 ± 19	0.106
Diagnostic methods				
Chest X-ray	143	135	132	
Normal	84 (51 %)	57 (38 %)	61 (39 %)	0.032
Infiltrate	13 (6.8 %)	17 (9.0 %)	22 (12 %)	0.248
Atelectasis	3 (1.8 %)	7 (4.6 %)	6 (3.8 %)	0.358
Pleural effusion	13 (7.8 %)	29 (19 %)	32 (20 %)	0.003
Pulmonary infarction	6 (3.6 %)	7 (4.6 %)	7 (4.5 %)	0.892
Vascular redistribution	12 (7.2 %)	8 (5.3 %)	13 (8.3 %)	0.572
Cardiomegaly	39 (24 %)	36 (24 %)	34 (22 %)	0.895
Electrocardiogram	156	142	133	
Normal	69 (42 %)	69 (45 %)	53 (34 %)	0.103
Atrial fibrillation	16 (9.6 %)	18 (12 %)	21 (13 %)	0.572
S1Q3T3 pattern	29 (18 %)	19 (13 %)	23 (15 %)	0.459
Negative T wave	35 (21 %)	18 (12 %)	20 (13 %)	0.040
Right bundle branch block	35 (17 %)	33 (16 %)	33 (18 %)	0.187
Thoracic CT scan	126	106	116	
High probability	126 (100 %)	106 (100 %)	116 (100 %)	–
Ventilation-perfusion lung scan	50	53	49	
High probability	49 (98 %)	46 (87 %)	46 (94 %)	0.224

VTE venous thromboembolism, *SBP* systolic blood pressure, *bpm* beats per minute, *PE* pulmonary embolism, *TKA* total knee arthroplasty, *THA* total hip arthroplasty

such patients had hypoxemia (Sat O_2 levels <90 %), one in every five patients had tachycardia (over 110 beats/min), and one in every eight patients had systolic hypotension (<100 mmHg). Dyspnea and hypoxemia were significantly more common in patients developing PE after hip fracture than in those undergoing TKA or THA.

Acute PE appeared significantly earlier in patients undergoing TKA (18 ± 8 days after surgery) than in those undergoing hip fracture (22 ± 19 days) or THA (27 ± 20 days). One in every two patients with PE (49 %) had a normal chest X-ray. In those with an abnormal chest X-ray, the most common findings were cardiomegaly (27 %), pleural effusion (18 %), or infiltrate (13 %). As for the electrocardiogram, it was normal in 44 % of patients with PE. The most common abnormalities were a right bundle branch block (23 %), a negative T wave (17 %), $S_1Q_3T_3$ pattern (16 %), or atrial fibrillation (13 %).

Table 4.3 Clinical characteristics of patients with deep vein thrombosis in the RIETE registry

	TKA	THA	Hip fracture	p value
Patients, N	147	155	130	
Initial VTE presentation				
Swelling	139 (95 %)	149 (96 %)	126 (98 %)	0.331
Pain	137 (95 %)	138 (89 %)	108 (84 %)	0.016
Proximal DVT	68 (47 %)	124 (82 %)	107 (84 %)	<0.001
Upper-extremity DVT	1 (0.7 %)	1 (0.6 %)	0	0.647
Time from surgery to DVT (days)	22 ± 18	31 ± 19	29 ± 21	0.070
Diagnostic methods				
Ultrasonography	147	155	130	
Thrombosis	132 (90 %)	151 (97 %)	128 (98 %)	0.055
Venography	15	4	2	
Thrombosis	15 (100 %)	4 (100 %)	2 (100 %)	–

DVT deep vein thrombosis, *TKA* total knee arthroplasty, *THA* total hip arthroplasty

Among 432 patients presenting with only DVT signs, the most common symptoms were swelling (96 %) and pain (89 %), as shown in Table 4.3. Pain was more commonly found in patients undergoing TKA (95 %) than in those undergoing THA (89 %) or hip fracture surgery (84 %). One in every three patients (31 %) presented with isolated distal DVT, and 69 % had proximal DVT. Distal DVT was more common in patients undergoing TKA (53 %) than in those undergoing THA (18 %) or hip fracture surgery (16 %). Only two patients (0.5 %) presented with upper-extremity DVT (secondary to an indwelling central venous catheter). Again, acute DVT appeared significantly earlier in patients undergoing TKA (22 ± 18 days after surgery) than in those undergoing hip fracture (29 ± 21 days) or THA (31 ± 19 days). All 432 patients underwent compression ultrasonography (CUS), which was negative in only 21 patients (4.9 %). Interestingly, it was positive in the 97 % of patients undergoing THA and 98 % of those undergoing surgery for hip fracture (98 %) but in "only" 90 % of those undergoing TKA.

Routine Screening for DVT After Major Joint Surgery

Since the vast majority of patients with DVT experience swelling or pain in the operated leg, the diagnosis of DVT by physical examination in patients operated on the hip or the knee is often equivocal. After surgery, many patients complain swelling and/or tenderness, and it is often difficult to decide whether symptoms or signs are caused by surgery itself or are associated with DVT.

Concern about the potential risk for PE as a result of undetected (and not treated) DVT has led clinicians to consider performing routine screening tests to diagnose asymptomatic DVT before hospital discharge. An extensive search including contrast venography would be costly and cause inconvenience to many patients. A non-invasive search for silent DVT using CUS would be a reasonable alternative, but it does not reliably detect asymptomatic DVT [6–11]. In fact, current guidelines from the American College of Chest Physicians (ACCP), based on evidence from these studies, recommend against the routine use of CUS screening at hospital discharge in asymptomatic patients following major joint surgery [12].

We hypothesized that a CUS search guided by physical examination could be more cost-effective [13]. We performed systematic physical examination before hospital discharge in a series of consecutive patients operated of major hip or knee surgery. Those with suspected DVT underwent bilateral CUS. It was a prospective, multicenter, and cohort study conducted between September 2003 and October 2004 in 43 Spanish hospitals. Consecutive patients operated because of TKA, THA, or hip fracture, who were available for a follow-up assessment 3 months after discharge, were eligible for the study. Patients received prophylaxis with low-molecular-weight heparin (LMWH) according to each center protocols. The circumferences of the two legs were measured at discharge at the ankle (at its minimum circumference) and the calf (at its maximum circumference). Those patients exhibiting over 2 cm of difference between both legs were considered to have suspected DVT and underwent bilateral CUS. Then, patients with no DVT identified at discharge underwent repeat physical examination on days 45 and 90 after surgery. If there was suspected DVT with the same clinical criteria as at discharge, CUS testing was performed to confirm the diagnosis.

During the study period, 1,033 patients were operated, TKA 410 patients, THA 393 patients, and hip fracture 230 patients. Their clinical characteristics are depicted in Table 4.4. Three patients developed acute, symptomatic, and objectively confirmed PE during admission (one died of PE). They all had sudden dyspnea with chest pain and no swelling in the legs. Five additional patients died. Routine examination for DVT was performed before discharge in the remaining 1,025 patients; in 105, (10 %) the findings of this examination suggested the presence of DVT. Of these, the diagnosis was confirmed by CUS in 24 (23 %), as shown in Table 4.5. The DVT was ipsilateral in 23 patients, bilateral in one. No patient had DVT in the asymptomatic leg. Of the 1,001 patients who were discharged with no DVT or PE, 978 (98 %) received LMWH prophylaxis for a few weeks after discharge.

From discharge to day 45, ten (1.0 %) patients died, 1 of them of PE (confirmed at necropsy). She started with persistent dyspnea shortly after discharge but had no suspected DVT at discharge. The cause of death for the remaining patients was identified in 5 (heart failure 2, infection 2, stroke 1), but 4 patients died at home due to an unknown cause. At day 45, fifty-nine (5.9 %) patients had suspected DVT, the diagnosis being confirmed by CUS in 17 (29 %). From day 45 to day 90, four (0.4 %) patients died (heart failure 2, stroke 1, unknown 2), and 2 patients had clinically overt PE (confirmed by lung scan). Fifty-three (5.5 %) patients had suspected DVT at day 90, diagnosis confirmed by CUS in 10 (19 %). The DVT was ipsilateral in 23 patients, contralateral in 3, and bilateral in one.

This prospective cohort study reveals that our limited diagnostic workup for DVT before discharge in patients operated of hip or knee surgery has the capacity to identify 44 % of the patients who will become symptomatic later. One in every

Table 4.4 Clinical characteristics of the patients, according to the type of surgery

Variables	Total knee replacement	Total hip replacement	Hip fracture
Patients			
Number	410	393	230
Mean age (years ± SD)	70 ± 7	67 ± 12	78 ± 13
Age (range)	39–85	23–100	22–97
Gender (males)	97 (24 %)	179 (46 %)	60 (26 %)
Body weight (kg ± SD)	76 ± 12	74 ± 13	67 ± 13
BMI > 25	345 (84 %)	290 (74 %)	115 (50 %)
Surgery			
Regional anesthesia	336 (82 %)	300 (76 %)	199 (87 %)
Surgery duration (min ± SD)	97 ± 27	103 ± 0.9	73 ± 31
Transfusion	403 (98 %)	389 (99 %)	224 (97 %)
Length of stay (days ± SD)	10 ± 19	10 ± 8	12 ± 25
LMWH prophylaxis	409 (99.8 %)	393 (100 %)	230 (100 %)
LMWH dose > 3,400 IU/day	408 (99 %)	388 (99 %)	225 (98 %)
Prophylaxis ≥ 3 weeks	332 (81 %)	315 (80 %)	178 (77 %)
Comorbid diseases			
Cancer	8 (2.0 %)	12 (3.1 %)	15 (6.5 %)
Ischemic heart disease	21 (5.1 %)	20 (5.1 %)	27 (12 %)
Chronic lung disease	32 (7.8 %)	45 (11 %)	17 (7.4 %)
Diabetes	73 (18 %)	57 (15 %)	52 (23 %)
Prior VTE	19 (4.6 %)	11 (2.8 %)	7 (3.0 %)

SD standard deviation, *BMI* body mass index, *LMWH* low-molecular-weight heparin, *IU* international units, *VTE* venous thromboembolism

Table 4.5 Incidence of symptomatic VTE and results of the workup study

	Discharge	Day 45	Day 90
Patients	1,033	990	965
Clinically overt PE	2 (0.2 %)	0	2 (0.2 %)
Fatal PE	1 (0.1 %)	1 (0.1 %)	0
Death, other reasons	4 (0.4 %)	9 (0.9 %)	4 (0.4 %)
Suspected DVT	105 (10 %)	59 (5.9 %)	53 (5.5 %)
CUS-confirmed DVT	24 (2.3 %)	17 (1.7 %)	10 (1.0 %)

PE pulmonary embolism, *DVT* deep vein thrombosis, *CUS* compression ultrasonography

ten patients had leg swelling identified by the screening strategy at discharge, 24 (2.3 % of the overall series) were diagnosed with proximal DVT. During follow-up, 112 additional patients had suspected DVT, 27 (2.6 %) were confirmed. However, our workup failed to detect three (0.3 %) episodes of symptomatic PE, of whom one patient died.

In conclusion, our limited diagnostic workup for DVT before discharge has the capacity to identify 44 % of those patients who will become symptomatic afterwards. A randomized controlled trial is necessary to confirm whether this strategy is of clinical benefit in daily practice.

Diagnosis Steps in Daily Practice

First step in diagnosis VTE is the suspicion. Acute venous thromboembolism should be suspected in patients with a combination of suggestive symptoms and/or signs. Most patients with confirmed PE do not have clinically evident DVT, and around 30 % of patients with symptomatic DVT have asymptomatic PE.

Suggestive symptoms and signs could include [14] the following :

- *DVT*: unilateral leg pain, swelling, tenderness, increased temperature, pitting edema, and prominent superficial veins
- *PE*: breathlessness, chest pain, hemoptysis, collapse, tachycardia, hypotension, tachypnea, raised jugular venous pressure, focal signs in chest, and hypoxia/cyanosis

Several diagnostic algorithms can be used to assess the clinical probability of having DVT and PE [14, 15]. Most commonly used are, probably, the Wells score for DVT and the revised Geneva score for PE (Table 4.6).

Moreover, it should be necessary to speak about D-dimer, which is a degradation product of cross-linked fibrin. D-dimer levels are elevated in plasma in the presence of an acute clot. Hence, a normal D-dimer level renders acute PE or DVT unlikely (the negative predictive value of D-dimer is high). On the other hand, although D-dimer is very specific for fibrin, the specificity of fibrin for VTE is poor because

Table 4.6 Probability scores for the assessment of suspected VTE

Wells score		Revised Geneva score	
Parameter	Score	Parameter	Score
Active cancer within last 6 months or palliative	1	Age 65 or over	1
Recently bedridden >3 days, or major surgery requiring regional or general anesthetic in past 4 weeks	1	Previous DVT/PE	3
Calf swelling >3 cm compared to other calf	1	Surgery or fracture (<1 month)	2
Collateral superficial veins (nonvaricose)	1	Active malignant condition	2
			3
Pitting edema (confined to symptomatic leg)	1	Unilateral lower limb pain	2
Swelling of entire leg	1	Hemoptysis	3
Localized pain along distribution of deep venous system	1	Heart rate:	5
		75–94 rpm	
		≥95 rpm	
Paralysis, paresis, or recent cast immobilization of lower extremities	1	Pain or deep palpation of lower limb or unilateral edema	4
Previously documented DVT	1		
Alternative diagnosis at least as likely	−2		
Probability of DVT		Probability of PE	
Low	0–1	Low (8 %)	0–3
Intermediate	2–6	Intermediate (28 %)	4–10
High	≥7	High (74 %)	11

fibrin is produced in a wide variety of conditions, such as postoperative period, and the positive predictive value of D-dimer is low [16]. Therefore, D-dimer is not useful for confirming VTE.

For confirmation of a clinically suspected VTE, we usually need an imaging test [14, 16].

- *Confirmation of a suspected DVT*: Venous ultrasound is the imaging investigation of choice for patients with suspected DVT. Patients who have a negative or inadequate initial scan, but who have a persisting clinical suspicion of DVT or whose symptoms do not settle, should have a repeat ultrasound scan at 5–7 days. The same recommendation is made for patients with a moderate suspicion with a positive D-dimer result or those whose, on clinical revision, suspicion of DVT remains high.
- *Confirmation of a suspected PE*: Computed tomography pulmonary angiography should be the first line investigation of pulmonary embolism, assessing the right ventricular/left ventricular ratio as an indicator of severity. Isotope lung scintigraphy should be considered if computed tomography pulmonary angiography is unavailable, and the patient is clinically stable.

Treatment

The objectives of VTE treatment are to improve acute symptoms and to prevent thrombus extension, early recurrence, and death from PE. In addition, treatment should prevent late recurrences and the development of long-term sequels such as postthrombotic syndrome and chronic pulmonary hypertension. In most patients, the initial treatment of DVT and PE is similar since both conditions are considered different manifestations of the same disease (VTE). Anticoagulation remains the mainstay of VTE treatment since the landmark study by Barritt and Jordan more than 50 years ago reporting a significant reduction in mortality and recurrences in patients with symptomatic PE treated with intravenous unfractionated heparin (UFH) and oral anticoagulants [17].

Initial Therapy

General Measures

Elevation of the legs and initial bed rest may provide relief of pain and tenderness in most patients with acute DVT. Although strict bed rest for a few days has been advocated for many years in combination with anticoagulation to prevent PE from dislodgement of the thrombus from the vein wall, recent evidence indicates that early ambulation does not increase the risk for PE and, in combination with com-

Table 4.7 Recommended dose regimens for LMWH and fondaparinux for VTE treatment

Agent	Dose
Enoxaparin	1.0 mg/kg BID or 1.5 mg/kg OD
Dalteparin	200 IU/kg OD
Tinzaparin	175 IU/kg OD
Nadroparin	4,100 IU BID if weight <50 kg
	6,150 IU BID if weight 50–70 kg
	9,200 IU BID if weight >70 kg
Bemiparin	115 IU/kg OD
Fondaparinux	5 mg OD if weight <50 kg
	7.5 mg if weight 50–100 kg
	10 mg if weight >100 kg

pression, improves leg symptoms [18–20]. The latest American College of Chest Physicians (ACCP) guidelines recommend early ambulation, when feasible, in preference to bed rest [21].

Anticoagulation

As mentioned above, anticoagulation represents the main therapy for both acute DVT and PE. During more than 30 years, the standard initial treatment consisted of intravenous UFH, adjusted to body weight, giving a bolus of 80 IU/kg followed by a continuous IV infusion, at doses adjusted to achieve an activated partial thromboplastin time (aPTT) within a therapeutic range 1.5–2.5 times the control time within the first 24 h. The reason for this need of monitoring of the anticoagulant effect is that UFH is a heterogeneous molecule, leading to unpredictable pharmacokinetics and a narrow therapeutic window. UFH may be administered also subcutaneously twice daily and also requires for monitoring for dose adjustment.

During the 1990s, low-molecular-weight heparins (LMWHs) were introduced for the treatment of VTE. These heparin fractions have a more favorable and predictable pharmacokinetic response than UFH when administered subcutaneously, and for that reason, do not require routine monitoring other than platelet count in most patients and are suitable for once or twice daily subcutaneous administration at doses adjusted to the patient's weight [21]. Regarding efficacy, several meta-analyses conclude that LMWHs are at least as effective as and more convenient than UFH for the initial treatment of VTE [22]. For these reasons, LMWHs have become the initial treatment of choice for DVT and most cases with PE. LMWH can be given once or twice daily for VTE treatment. A meta-analysis including data from five trials shows a nonsignificant reduction in the VTE recurrences and bleeding complications in patients receiving a single daily dose [23]. The recommended doses and regimens of LMWH used in the treatment of VTE are shown in Table 4.7.

Some trials have evaluated the possibility of treating VTE patients with LMWH at home. There is consistent evidence that outpatient treatment of DVT and for selected patients with PE is effective, safe, and cost saving [24].

Fondaparinux, a synthetic indirect selective inhibitor of factor Xa, has also been evaluated in the treatment of VTE, showing similar efficacy and safety as LMWH, without the need for monitoring. The doses are 5, 7.5, and 10 mg once daily depending on the patient's weight and are given by subcutaneous injection. For patients with a weight between 50 and 100 kg, the daily dose is 7.5 mg [25, 26].

Patients with DVT or PE should be treated with any of the aforementioned anti-coagulants once the diagnosis is confirmed by objective diagnostic tests. Nevertheless, treatment should be started until the diagnosis is confirmed if the clinical suspicion is very high.

Initial treatment with UFH, LMWH, or fondaparinux should be continued for 5–7 days [21]. Current recommendation is to start both heparin, LMWH, or fonda-parinux and oral vitamin K antagonists (VKA) at the time of diagnosis and to dis-continue parenteral anticoagulants after 5 days once the international normalized ratio (INR) is higher than 2–0 for at least 24 h. Warfarin, which is one of the most commonly used VKA drugs for VTE management, is usually started at a dose of 5–10 mg, depending on the age and health status of patients. Subsequent doses should be adjusted to keep the INR around 2.5 (2.0–3.0). Some selected patients (such as those in whom oral VKA are contraindicated for patients, pregnant women, or patients with active cancer) should receive LMWH as secondary prevention for recurrent VTE [27]. The duration of anticoagulation for most VTE cases is at least 3 months and will be addressed in more detail in another section of this chapter.

Thrombolysis

The natural process of plasmin degradation of fibrin in the thrombus is slow, and there-fore, damage to the venous valves in the legs may occur. For this reason, some studies have assessed the role of systemic and catheter-directed thrombolytic (CDT) therapy in patients with acute massive proximal DVT (phlegmasia) with the goals of avoiding venous ischemia, reducing acute symptoms, and the risk of postthrombotic syndrome (PTS). A review of 12 studies showed a 66 % risk reduction of PTS on long-term fol-low-up from 65 % with standard anticoagulation to 48 % with anticoagulation and systemic thrombolysis [28]. The problem is that the risk of major bleeding, including stroke, increased (RR 1.73). For that reason, CDT has been evaluated and shown to be a promising alternative, as shown in a recent trial where CDT increased the 6-month iliofemoral patency rate from 36 to 64 % without a significant increase in bleeding complications [29]. Current indications for CDT include patients with massive DVT causing circulatory limb threat, patients who have not achieved therapeutic objectives with initial anticoagulation, and in selected patients with acute iliofemoral DVT [30].

Vena Cava Filters

The objective of inferior vena cava partial interruption using filters is to prevent pulmonary embolism in patients with DVT. Insertion of an inferior vena cava

Table 4.8 Contraindications for anticoagulant treatment in patients with VTE

Absolute
  Intracranial bleeding
  Severe active bleeding
  Recent brain, eye, or spinal surgery
  Malignant hypertension
Relative
  Recent major surgery
  Recent large thromboembolic stroke
  Active gastrointestinal tract bleeding
  Severe hypertension
  Severe renal or hepatic failure
  Thrombocytopenia (<50,000/ml)

filter (IVCF) is currently indicated for patients with acute VTE and a contraindication to receive anticoagulant treatment and for patients with recurrent VTE despite adequate anticoagulation therapy. Table 4.8 shows the main contraindications for anticoagulation. Although IVCF prevent clinically relevant PE in patients with DVT, they increase the risk of recurrent DVT up to 2 years after insertion from 12 to 21 % [31]. For that reason, removable filters should be considered when possible. For patients with VTE who have received a filter because anticoagulation was contraindicated, anticoagulation is recommended once the bleeding risk resolves [21].

Long-Term Treatment (Secondary Prevention)

After the initial therapy for 5–10 days, extended anticoagulation is required to prevent thrombus extension and recurrent VTE. The most frequently used agents for long-term anticoagulation or secondary prevention are oral VKAs such as warfarin or acenocoumarol. Due to delayed onset of their anticoagulant action, VKA should be initiated at the same time as heparins and overlap them for at least 5–7 days, targeting international normalized ratio (INR) of 2.5 (2.0–3.0) [21]. Once INR is higher than 2.0 for more than 24 h, heparins may be discontinued. The usual starting dose of warfarin is 5–10 mg, although the latter is faster, achieving a therapeutic INR by the fifth day of treatment.

Several trials have evaluated the use of subcutaneous LMWH for the long-term treatment of VTE. The results of these studies show that fixed or weight-adjusted LMWHs are at least as effective as INR-adjusted VKA and probably safer [32]. Although heparins need daily subcutaneous injections, they have the advantage of the lack of monitoring, other than periodic platelet count. Some studies have shown that in cancer patients with VTE, LMWHs are more effective and equally safe than VKA [27, 33]. The recommended dosing regimens for these agents are dalteparin 200 U/kg daily for 1 month, followed by 150 U/kg for at least 5 months or tinzaparin 175 U/kg once daily for at least 6 months.

Table 4.9 ACCP recommendation for the duration of anticoagulant therapy

Patient characteristics	Recommended duration	Grade
DVT secondary to a reversible risk factor	3 months	1A
First unprovoked DVT	At least 3 months	1A
First unprovoked proximal DVT and low risk for bleeding and good anticoagulant monitoring	Longer than 3 months	1A
Second episode of unprovoked VTE	Long-term treatment	1A
First episode of unprovoked isolated distal DVT	3 months	2B
DVT and cancer	3–6 months with LMWH and then indefinitely or until cancer resolves	1C

Duration of Anticoagulation

The optimal duration of anticoagulant treatment of VTE remains controversial, since the reduction in the incidence or recurrent thrombosis achieved by prolonged therapy should be weighed against the risk for bleeding complications. Two factors are determinant for the risk of recurrent VTE after the discontinuation of treatment: how adequate was the anticoagulation in the initial phase and whether the VTE at presentation was idiopathic (unprovoked) or related to the presence of risk factors (transient or permanent). Interestingly, the form of VTE presentation influences the type of recurrence, as it has been observed that patients presenting with PE are more likely to recur with another PE, and patients with DVT usually recur with a DVT.

Prolonged anticoagulation is very effective in preventing recurrent VTE; however, this benefit is offset by the risk of major bleeding, which is between 1 and 3 % per year. The 8th ACCP guidelines recommend anticoagulation to be continued for at least 3 months for patients with a first episode of idiopathic proximal DVT or PE and without excessive bleeding risk [21]. The current recommendations for duration of therapy in different clinical scenarios are shown in Table 4.9.

The duration of secondary prevention in patients with a first episode of unprovoked VTE who have a low risk for bleeding needs to be established due to its enormous clinical and economic impact, since this group represents between 25 and 50 % of patients with VTE. Therefore, there is an increasing interest in the use of clinical prognostic factors to help physicians deciding the optimal duration of anticoagulant treatment. The presence of elevated levels of D-dimer (DD) and the presence of residual DVT assessed by compression ultrasonography after cessation of treatment have been associated with an increased risk of recurrent VTE and might be useful influence in the decision to prolong treatment. One study from Italy showed that the risk of VTE recurrence in patients with normal DD levels 1 month after discontinuation of anticoagulation and with abnormal levels at 3 months and thereafter is higher than in those with normal DD levels at the third month and afterward [34]. Another study from the same group of investigators included patients with unprovoked VTE who underwent DD testing 1 month after oral anticoagulant discontinuation [35]. Patients with normal DD did not resume anticoagulation, whereas those with abnormal DD were randomized to resume or discontinue treatment. The rate of VTE recurrences was 2.9 and 15 %, respectively.

A recent trial included patients with a first episode of proximal DVT, who were randomized after an uneventful 3-month period of anticoagulation to receive fixed-duration anticoagulation (no further treatment for secondary thrombosis and an additional period of 3 months for unprovoked DVT) or flexible-duration, ultrasound-guided anticoagulation (no further anticoagulation for patients with recanalized veins and continued treatment in all other patients) [36]. The rate of recurrent VTE was 17 and 12 % for patients allocated to fixed and flexible-duration anticoagulation, respectively. The role of these parameters in guiding clinical decision about the duration of treatment remains uncertain and further trials are needed.

Graduated Elastic Stocking

Brandjes and coworkers reported in 1997 that the use of knee-length 30–40-mmHg stockings for at least 2 years in patients with symptomatic proximal DVT reduced the risk of development of postthrombotic syndrome (PTS) by 50 % [37]. Further evidence to support the use of stockings to prevent PTS was provided by another study where the investigators also found a 50 % reduction in the incidence of PTS after 2 years [38]. The current ACCP guidelines recommend stockings (30–40 mmHg at the ankle) started as soon as possible and continued for a minimum of 2 years or longer if patients develop symptoms of PTS [21].

New Anticoagulants (See Also Chap. 6)

Current treatment of VTE has a number of limitations: need for parenteral heparins initially, frequent laboratory monitoring, and dose adjustment of oral vitamin K antagonists, which also have frequent food and drug interactions. For these reasons, there has been intensive research to develop an oral anticoagulant that does not require laboratory monitoring and with a good efficacy-safety profile during the acute and long-term phase of VTE treatment. Phase III trials have been completed with two direct factor Xa inhibitors (rivaroxaban and apixaban) and with a direct thrombin inhibitor (dabigatran).

In an open-label randomized noninferiority trial, oral rivaroxaban (15 mg twice daily for 3 weeks followed by 20 mg once daily) was compared with subcutaneous enoxaparin followed by vitamin K antagonists (VKA) for 3, 6, or 12 months in patients with acute symptomatic proximal DVT. In parallel, the authors conducted a double-blind, randomized, and superiority study comparing rivaroxaban alone (20 mg once daily) with placebo for an additional 6 or 12 months in patients who had completed 6–12 months of treatment for DVT or PE [39]. In the acute DVT study, recurrent symptomatic VTE was reported in 2.1 % of patients receiving rivaroxaban and 3.0 % in those receiving enoxaparin and VKA ($p < 0.001$ for noninferiority). Major or clinically relevant bleeding occurred in 8.1 % of patients in both groups. In the continued treatment study, recurrent VTE occurred in 1.3 % of the rivaroxaban group, compared to 7.1 % in the placebo group ($p < 0.001$), which represents an 82 % risk reduction. On the other hand, major bleeding occurred in 0.7 and 0 %, respectively ($p = 0.11$). In summary, this oral anticoagulant, used at fixed doses and without the need for monitoring, may provide an effective and safe single-drug approach for the initial and long-term treatment of VTE.

In a randomized, double-blind, and noninferiority trial, patients with acute VTE treated initially with heparin or LMWH for a median of 9 days were randomized to receive oral dabigatran (150 mg twice daily) with warfarin at doses adjusted to achieve an INR of 2.0–3.0 [40]. Both oral agents were given for 6 months. During that period, recurrent VTE occurred in 2.4 % of patients receiving secondary prevention with dabigatran and in 2.1 % of those receiving warfarin ($p < 0.001$ for noninferiority). Major bleeding occurred in 1.6 and 1.9 % of patients, respectively (hazard ratio 0.82; 95 % CI, 0.45–1.48). This study shows that a fixed oral dose of dabigatran is as effective and safe as warfarin for the secondary prevention of VTE after an initial period of at least 5 days of heparin or LMWH.

References

1. Guijarro R, Montes J, San Román C, Arcelus JI, Barillari G, Granero X, Monreal M. Venous thromboembolism and bleeding after total knee and hip arthroplasty. Findings from the Spanish National Discharge Database. Thromb Haemost. 2011;105:610–5.
2. Arcelus JI, Caprini JA, Monreal M, Suárez C, González-Fajardo J. The management and outcome of acute venous thromboembolism: a prospective registry including 4011 patients. J Vasc Surg. 2003;38:916–22.
3. Laporte S, Mismetti P, Découssus H, Uresandi F, Otero R, Lobo JL, Monreal M, RIETE Investigators. Clinical predictors for fatal pulmonary embolism in 15,520 patients with venous thromboembolism; findings from the registro informatizado de la enfermedad tromboembólica venosa (RIETE) Registry. Circulation. 2008;117:1711–6.
4. Arcelus JI, Monreal M, Caprini JA, Guisado JG, Soto MJ, Núñez MJ, Alvárez JC. Clinical presentation and time-course of postoperative venous thromboembolism. Findings from the RIETE Registry. Thromb Haemost. 2008;99:546–51.
5. www.riete.org. Accessed on 2 May 2011.
6. Wells PS, Lensing AWA, Davidson BL, Prins MH, Hirsh J. Accuracy of ultrasound for diagnosis of deep venous thrombosis in asymptomatic patients after orthopedic surgery. A meta-analysis. Ann Intern Med. 1995;122:47–53.
7. Robinson KS, Anderson DR, Gross M, Petrie D, Leighton R, Stanish W, Alexander D, Mitchell M, Flemming B, Gent M. Ultrasonographic screening before hospital discharge for deep venous thrombosis after arthroplasty: the post-arthroplasty screening study. A randomized, controlled trial. Ann Intern Med. 1997;127:439–45.
8. Leclerc JR, Gent M, Hirsh J, Geerts WH, Ginsberg JS, for the Canadian Collaborative Group. The incidence of symptomatic venous thromboembolism during and after prophylaxis with enoxaparin. A multi-institutional cohort study of patients who underwent hip or knee arthroplasty. Arch Intern Med. 1998;158:873–8.

9. Verlato F, Bruchi O, Prandoni P, Camporese G, Maso G, Busonera F, Girolami A, Andreozzi GM, for the WODOS Investigators Group. The value of ultrasound screening for proximal vein thrombosis after total hip arthroplasty. A prospective cohort study. Thromb Haemost. 2001;86:534–7.
10. Schmidt B, Michler R, Klein M, Faulmann G, Weber C, Schellong S. Ultrasound screening for distal vein thrombosis is not beneficial after major orthopedic surgery. A randomized controlled trial. Thromb Haemost. 2003;90:949–54.
11. Schellong SM, Beyer J, Kakkar AK, Halbritter K, Eriksson BI, Turpie AGG, Misselwitz F, Kälebo P. Ultrasound screening for asymptomatic deep vein thrombosis after major orthopaedic surgery: the VENUS study. J Thromb Haemost. 2007;5:14311437.
12. Geerts WH, Bergqvist D, Pineo GF, Heit JA, Samama CM, Lassen MR, Colwell W. Prevention of venous thromboembolism. American college of chest physicians evidence-based clinical practice guidelines (8th edition). Chest. 2008;133:381S–453.
13. Monreal M, Peidro L, Resines C, Garcés C, Fernández JL, Garagorri E, González JC, NETCOT Investigators. Limited diagnostic workup for deep vein thrombosis after major joint surgery: findings from a prospective, multicentre, cohort study. Thromb Haemost. 2008;99:1112–5.
14. Scottish Intercollegiate Guidelines Network (SIGN). Prevention and management of venous thromboembolism. 2010; Edinburgh.
15. Wells PS, Anderson DR, Rodger M, Ginsberg JS, Kearon C, Gent M, et al. Derivation of a simple clinical model to categorize patients probability of pulmonary embolism: increasing the models utility with the SimpliRED D-dimer. Thromb Haemost. 2000;83:416–20.
16. Torbicky A, Perrier A, Konstantinides S, Agnelli G, Gallie N, Pruszczyk P, et al. Guidelines on the diagnosis and management of acute pulmonary embolism. Eur Heart J. 2008;29:2276–315.
17. Barritt DW, Jordan SC. Anticoagulant drugs in the treatment of pulmonary embolism: a controlled trial. Lancet. 1960;i:1309–12.
18. Aschwanden M, Labs KH, Engel H, et al. Acute deep vein thrombosis: early mobilization does not increase the frequency of pulmonary embolism. Thromb Haemost. 2001;85:42–6.
19. Trujillo-Santos J, Perea-Milla E, Jimenez-Puente A, et al. Bed rest or ambulation in the initial treatment of patients with acute deep vein thrombosis or pulmonary embolism: findings from the RIETE registry. Chest. 2005;127:1631–6.
20. Partsch H, Blattler W. Compression and walking versus bed rest in the treatment of proximal deep venous thrombosis with low molecular weight heparin. J Vasc Surg. 2000;32:861–9.
21. Kearon C, Kahn SR, Agnelli G, et al. Antithrombotic therapy for venous thromboembolic disease: American college of chest physicians evidence-based clinical practice guidelines (8th edition). Chest. 2008;133:454–545.
22. Dolovich LR, Ginsberg JS, Douketis JD, Holbrook AM, Cheah G. A meta-analysis comparing low-molecular-weight heparins with unfractionated heparin in the treatment of venous thromboembolism. Arch Intern Med. 2000;24:181–8.
23. Van Dogen CJ, MacGillavry MR, Prins MH. Once versus twice daily LMWH for the initial treatment of venous thromboembolism. Cochrane Database Syst Rev. 2005;(3):CD003074.
24. Othieno R, Abu Affan M, Okpo E. Home versus in-patient treatment for deep vein thrombosis. Cochrane Database Syst Rev. 2007;(3):CD003076.
25. Büller HR, Davidson B, Decousus H, et al. Fondaparinux or enoxaparin for the initial treatment of symptomatic deep venous thrombosis. A randomized trial. Ann Intern Med. 2004;140:867–73.
26. Matisse Investigators. Subcutaneous fondaparinux versus intravenous unfractionated heparin in the initial treatment of pulmonary embolism. N Engl J Med. 2003;349:1695–702.
27. Lee A, Levine M, Naker R, et al. Low molecular weight heparin versus a coumarin for the prevention of recurrent venous thromboembolism in patients with cancer. N Engl J Med. 2003;349:146–53.
28. Watson LI, Armon MP. Thrombolysis for acute deep vein thrombosis. Cochrane Database Syst Rev. 2004;(4):CD002783.

29. Enden T, Klow N-E, Sandvik L, et al. Catheter-directed thrombolysis versus anticoagulant therapy alone in deep vein thrombosis: results of an open randomized, controlled trial reporting on short term patency. J Thromb Haemost. 2009;7:1268–75.
30. Vendantham S. Catheter-directed thrombolysis for deep vein thrombosis. Curr Opin Hematol. 2010;17:464–8.
31. Decousus H, Leizorovicz A, Parent F, et al. A clinical trial of vena cava filters in the prevention of pulmonary embolism in patients with proximal deep-vein thrombosis. N Engl J Med. 1998;338:409–16.
32. Iorio A, Guercini F, Pini M. Low-molecular-weight heparin for the long-term treatment of symptomatic venous thromboembolism: meta-analysis of the randomized comparisons with oral anticoagulants. J Thromb Haemost. 2003;1:1906–13.
33. Hull R, Pineo G, Brant R, et al. Long-term low-molecular-weight heparin versus usual care in proximal vein thrombosis patients with cancer. Am J Med. 2006;119:1062–72.
34. Cosmi B, Legnani C, Tosetto A, et al. Usefulness of repeated D-dimer testing after stopping anticoagulation for a first episode of unprovoked venous thromboembolism: the PROLONG II prospective study. Blood. 2010;115:481–8.
35. Palareti G, Cosmi B, Legnani C, et al. D-dimer testing to determine the duration of anticoagulant therapy. N Engl J Med. 2006;355:1780–9.
36. Prandoni P, Prins MH, Lensing AW, et al. Residual vein thrombosis to guide the duration of anticoagulation I patients with deep venous thrombosis: a randomized trial. Ann Intern Med. 2009;150:577–85.
37. Brandjes DP, Büller HR, Heijboer H, et al. Randomised trial of effect of compression stockings in patients with symptomatic proximal-vein thrombosis. Lancet. 1997;349:759–62.
38. Prandoni P, Lensing AW, Prins MH, et al. Below-knee stockings elastic compression stockings to prevent the post-thrombotic syndrome: a randomized, controlled trial. Ann Intern Med. 2004;141:249–56.
39. The EINSTEIN Investigators. Oral rivaroxaban for symptomatic venous thromboembolism. N Engl J Med. 2010;363:2499–510.
40. Schulman S, Kearon C, Kakkar AK, et al. Dabigatran versus warfarin in the treatment of acute venous thromboembolism. N Engl J Med. 2009;361:2342–52.

Chapter 5
Drugs for Thromboprophylaxis: Unfractionated Heparin, Low Molecular Weight Heparin, Warfarin, and Fondaparinux

José Aguirre and Alain Borgeat

Abstract The world of antithrombotic prophylaxis is a revolutionary phase due to the introduction of numerous new compounds in the daily practice. However, traditional antithrombotics are still in use. This chapter deals with advantages and disadvantages of the traditional drugs used in this context: unfractionated heparin, low molecular weight heparin, and fondaparinux. The use of these drugs will decrease, but specific indications will remain. This point will also be emphasized in this chapter.

Keywords Antithrombotic drugs • Unfractionated heparin • Low molecular weight heparin • Warfarin • Fondaparinux • Deep venous thrombosis • Pulmonary embolism

Introduction

The most widely available, approved, and currently used anticoagulants are unfractionated heparin (UFH), low molecular weight heparins (LMWHs) (e.g., enoxaparin, tinzaparin, dalteparin), vitamin K antagonists (VKA) (e.g., warfarin), and fondaparinux [1–3].

UFH has been discovered as animal-derived extractive drug in 1916 by Jay McLean at John Hopkins in Baltimore and has been available for nearly a century. Karl Paul Link discovered in 1940 coumarin as a substance contained in sweet clover hay which killed cattle by bleeding [4]. From the 1980s to the late 1990s, the evolution of UFH

J. Aguirre, M.D. • A. Borgeat, M.D.(✉)
Division of Anesthesiology, Balgrist University Hospital,
Forchstrasse 340, 8008 Zürich, Switzerland
e-mail: alain.borgeat@balgrist.ch

J.V. Llau (ed.), *Thromboembolism in Orthopedic Surgery*,
DOI 10.1007/978-1-4471-4336-9_5, © Springer-Verlag London 2013

toward the chemically fractionated low molecular weight heparins and after further fractionating toward fondaparinux which contains the essential pentasaccharide anticoagulant structure shared by both UFH and LMWHs took place [4].

Patients undergoing major orthopedic surgery are subjected to the risk of venous thromboembolism (VTE), consisting in deep venous thrombosis (DVT) and pulmonary embolism (PE), independently of the choice of anesthesia. Without thromboprophylaxis, 40–60 % of patients will develop DVT, and 10 % of those will suffer a PE [5, 6]. After total hip arthroplasty and total knee arthroplasty, the prevalences of total DVT and PE are 41–85 % and ≤30 %, respectively [7–10]. Actually, the incidence of fatal PE is 0.1–0.2 with 480,000 VTE-related deaths estimated to occur annually in the EU [11].

Prophylaxis with coumarins has been the gold standard for VTE prevention after acute coronary syndrome for over 60 years. However, this treatment requires frequent monitoring for dose adjustment, and multiple interactions with other drugs are the major drawbacks of this drug. In the 1970s, VTE prevention after major surgery was started with heparins reducing postoperative VTE-related mortality to 5 %. Due to the need for aPTT monitoring for dosage adjustment, low molecular weight heparins (LMWH) were introduced 10 years later. Fondaparinux was the next development to hit the market, an effective and safe indirect factor-Xa inhibitor which is used parenterally [12].

The Use of Anticoagulants and Neuraxial Anesthesia

Neuraxial anesthesia bears the risk of spinal/epidural hematoma (SEH) with possible compression in the spinal canal, potentially resulting in neuroplegia if not recognized and treated early. The risk of SEH is about 1:150,000 but increases by 15-fold with the use of anticoagulant therapy without appropriate precautions [5]. This risk is further increased if indwelling epidural catheters are used. This requires a proper management of anticoagulated patients, particularly with the continuing development of new and possibly more potent anticoagulants. The risk of hematoma associated with a specific anticoagulant is difficult to estimate, and prospective randomized trials are not possible [13–15]. Therefore, a rigid strategy to balance the risk of hematoma with effective thromboprophylaxis is needed. Several national guidelines have been published, most of them based on case reports or pharmacokinetic properties of the most used agents, leading to drug-specific recommendations [5, 16]. Patient management focuses on the timing of needle/catheter placement and catheter removal according to the timing of anticoagulant drug administration. The goal is to perform these manipulations when the drug concentration is at its lowest [13–15]. Another strategy is to delay the initiation of postsurgical anticoagulation to further reduce the risk of hematoma [5]. However, the risk of hematoma is increased with concomitant use of medications such as nonsteroidal anti-inflammatory drugs or other anticoagulants, further complicating patient management. Therefore, all patients undergoing neuraxial anesthesia must be monitored for clinical signs of neurologic impairment to assure prompt intervention to avoid irreversible neurological complications [13–15].

Unfractionated Heparin

The anticoagulant action of UFH derives from the binding to antithrombin and catalyzing the inactivation of factors IIa, Xa, IXa, and, also if to a lesser extent, also from XIa and XIIa [5]. UFH binds to a number of plasma proteins of endothelial cells, macrophages, and platelet factor 4. This widespread binding leads to a low bioavailability and clinically unpredictable pharmacokinetic and pharmacodynamic properties. Moreover, it has also been associated with the occurrence of heparin-induced thrombocytopenia (HIT). UFH was clinically used from the 1970s onward and was the first anticoagulant to be used for the prevention and treatment of DVT and PE.

UFH has a short half-life (2–4 h) and a quick onset; therefore, they are considered to be safe and well controllable for thromboembolic prophylaxis and acute treatment of thrombosis. UFH has a number of limitations such as parenteral administration and possible development of life-threatening heparin-induced thrombocytopenia (HIT) type II (Table 5.1) [20, 21]. UFH requires laboratory monitoring, dosage adjustment, and potentially monitoring for HIT [22]. Due to its considerable intra- and interindividual variability, therapy with UFH is unpredictable and inappropriate for long-term use. One important advantage compared to LMWH is the possibility to neutralize its effect by protamine sulfate (Tables 5.2 and 5.3).

Unfractionated Heparin and Neuraxial Anesthesia

The consensus statement from the American Society of Regional Anesthesia and Pain Medicine (ASRA) on regional anesthesia in the anticoagulated patient bases its recommendations for UFH on the first recommendations more than 20 years ago which were supported by reviews of case series and case reports of postpuncture spinal hematoma [13–15]. ASRA recommends that UFH administration be delayed for 1 h after needle placement. Indwelling neuraxial catheters should be removed 2–4 h after the last UFH dose, and the next dose can be given 1 h after catheter removal. Notwithstanding, patients must be carefully monitored for any clinical signs of spinal hematoma [13–15].

Low Molecular Weight Heparin

LMWHs (e.g., enoxaparin, tinzaparin, dalteparin) are derived from UFH by enzymatic or chemical depolymerization and have therefore shorter heparin chains. This leads to a better bioavailability and therefore better predictability of effect without

Table 5.1 Advantages and disadvantages of anticoagulant therapy with warfarin, unfractionated heparin, low molecular weight heparin, and fondaparinux [17–19]

Anticoagulant	Advantages	Disadvantages
Warfarin	Gold standard for primary and secondary prophylaxis of venous thromboembolism	Frequent monitoring
	Oral administration	Slow onset and offset of action
	Can be antagonized with vitamin K	Drug and dietary interactions
		Narrow therapeutic window
		Risk of bleeding complications
UFH	Fast acting	Frequent monitoring
	High efficacy	Parenteral administration
	Fine regulation of dosage steps	Indirect action: needs antithrombin
	Antagonization with protamine sulfate	Potential of severe heparin-induced thrombocytopenia
		Nonspecific protein binding with unpredictable response
		Variable bioavailability
		Risk of bleeding complications
		Risk of osteoporosis
LMWH	Variable dosage: once or twice daily	Subcutaneous injection
	High efficacy	Indirect action: needs antithrombin
	No monitoring needed (if no renal insufficiency)	Risk of thrombocytopenia
		Risk of osteoporosis
		Bleeding complications (in patients with renal insufficiency)
Fondaparinux	Once-daily dose	Subcutaneous injection
	Does not affect thrombin activity	Indirect action: needs antithrombin
	Inhibits free factor Xa	
	Low risk of induced thrombocytopenia	
	No monitoring needed if no renal insufficiency	

the need for routine monitoring, if there is no renal insufficiency. In this case and due to half-life prolongation, monitoring and dose reduction are recommended [22]. LMWH also binds to antithrombin and shows a selective inhibitory effect on factor Xa [22]. LMWH has greater inhibitory activity against factor Xa than thrombin (IIa), and the protein binding of these agents is less than that of UFH. Consequently, the risk of HIT is therefore lower, and the anticoagulation is more predictable compared to UFH. LMHW is contraindicated in patients with a creatinine clearance of <30 ml/min. The longer half-life of LMWH (2–6 h after single sc injection) allows different dosage regimens: once daily for thromboembolic prophylaxis or twice daily for treatment of thrombosis [23].

LMWHs have overcome some of the limitations of UFH such as a more predictable anticoagulant with no need for routine coagulation monitoring. The need for subcutaneous administration has some limits in the use for the outpatient setting.

Table 5.2 Comparison of advantages or disadvantages of different anticoagulants and their clinical implications

Advantage or disadvantage of anticoagulants	Clinical implications
LMWH vs. UFH	
+ Increased bioavailability	Subcutaneous dosage possible
+ Inferior binding to plasma proteins	Predictable anticoagulant response, no monitoring needed
+ Inferior binding to platelet factor 4	Reduced risk of induced thrombocytopenia
+ Inferior binding to endothelium	Increased half-life with possible once-daily dosage
+ Inferior binding to bone cells	Reduced risk of osteoporosis
− Protamine sulfate as antidote less effective	Reduced reversal possibility after overdose or bleeding
Fondaparinux vs. LMHW	
+ Higher safety	No biological contamination, reduced risk of osteoporosis and of induced thrombocytopenia
+ Defined, single target (factor Xa)	Reduced vulnerability to interactions
− Inhibition of factor Xa less potent than heparin	Increased risk of thrombosis in acute coronary syndrome without the concomitant administration of heparin
− No antidote	Reduced reversal possibility after overdose or bleeding
Vitamin K antagonists vs. LMWH and fondaparinux	
+ Oral administration	Ideal for outpatient setting
+ Vitamin K as antidote	Reversal possible in case of overdose or bleeding
− Longer plasma half-life	Reduced reversal onset in case of overdose or bleeding
− Interaction with drugs, food, and genetic polymorphisms	Close laboratory monitoring and dose adjustment

UFH unfractionated heparin, *LMWH* low molecular weight heparin

In summary, the advantages of LMWH over UFH are higher availability and longer half-life, which allow once-daily subcutaneous administration, more predictable anticoagulant responses that obviate the need of laboratory monitoring (for dosage tailoring), and less binding to platelet factor 4 and bone cells that results in a lower risk for thrombocytopenia and osteoporosis (Tables 5.2 and 5.3).

LMWH and Neuraxial Anesthesia

- *Preoperative LMWH*: ASRA recommends that needle placement should occur at least 10–12 h after the last dose of LMWH [13–15]. However, most European guidelines recommend a delay of at least 12 h, but a delay of 20 h is recommended by French guidelines [5]. ASRA further recommends that needle placement occurs at least 24 h after the last dose if a higher dose of LMWH is used

Table 5.3 Pharmacokinetic and pharmacodynamic characteristics of traditional and newer anticoagulants

	UFH	LMWH	Warfarin	Fondaparinux
Target	Factor Xa and thrombin	Factor Xa and thrombin	Vitamin K-dependent factors and inhibitors	Factor Xa
Source	Biological	Biological	Synthetic	Synthetic
Administration	IV/sc	Sc	Oral	Sc
Bioavailability	30 %	90 %	90 %	100 %
Half-life	1 h	4 h	15–44 h	17 h
Antidote	Protamine sulfate	Protamine sulfate	Vitamin K/FFP/PCC	No
Thrombocytopenia	<5 %	<1 %	No	?

FFP fresh frozen plasma, *PTCC* prothrombin complex concentrates, *IV* intravenous, *Sc* subcutaneous

(e.g., 1 mg/kg enoxaparin every 12 h or 1.5 mg/kg daily) [13–15]. Neuraxial techniques should be avoided in patients administered LMWH 2 h preoperatively due to coincidence with peak anticoagulant activity [13–15].

- *Postoperative LMWH*: Postoperative LMWH application is based on the dosing regimen chosen. Twice-daily administration might be associated with an increased risk of spinal hematoma [13–15]. The ASRA guidelines recommend that the first dose be administered at earliest 24 h postoperatively, independently of anesthetic technique, and only in the presence of correct surgical hemostasis. Indwelling catheters should be removed if indicated before initiation of LMWH therapy. In the case of epidural catheter, the indwelling catheter may be left overnight and removed the following day, with the first dose of LMWH administered at least 2 h after catheter removal [13–15]. If given once daily, the first postoperative LMWH dose should be administered 6–8 h postoperatively, and the second postoperative dose should occur not before 24 h after the first dose. Indwelling neuraxial catheters may be safely maintained, but the catheter should be removed 10–12 h after the last dose of LMWH. A further dose might be given 2 h after catheter removal. However, European guidelines recommend in this context a 4–6-h delay [5].

Vitamin K Antagonists

Long-term anticoagulation is still performed with VKA. Warfarin is the most frequently used. VKA interferes with the metabolism of vitamin K by influencing the posttranslational carboxylation of coagulation factors II, VII, IX, and X and other coagulation proteins such as proteins C, S, and Z, leading to a reduced coagulant effect by abolishing their potential to be activated on phospholipid surfaces after calcium-dependent binding [24]. The benefits of warfarin therapy in a wide range of patients with thromboembolic complications are well established. Hart et al. described in a meta-analysis of trials involving 2,900 patients that dose-adjusted warfarin reduced the relative risk of stroke by 62 % compared with placebo in patients with atrial fibrillation [25]. Nevertheless, warfarin has unpredictable pharmacodynamic, pharmacokinetic, and pharmacogenetic properties, causing major variability in patients' dose responses [24]. However, warfarin's use is hampered by numerous limitations like its narrow therapeutic window, its need for frequent coagulation monitoring and dose adjustments, dietary restrictions, bleeding risk, its delayed onset and offset of action, and frequent interactions with other drugs [26]. These problems lead to adverse effects, which might be responsible for additional hospitalizations (see Table 5.3) [27]. At the beginning, VKA therapy requires frequent therapeutic monitoring and dose adjustments using the international normalized ratio (INR), based on the prothrombin time (PT) [24]. Administration of vitamin K is recommended to reverse a mildly increased INR. In the case of life-threatening bleeding or intracranial hemorrhage, prothrombin complex concentrates are recommended [24, 28]. If prothrombin complex concentrates are not available, fresh frozen plasma is still used. Off-label use of recombinant factor VIIa has also been reported to reverse the INR effect [29].

VKA and Neuraxial Anesthesia

The anesthetic management of patients receiving warfarin for long-term therapy or as perioperative thromboembolic prophylaxis is controversially discussed. The ASRA consensus statement bases its recommendations mainly on case reports of spinal hematoma, drug pharmacology, and on the clinical relevance of vitamin K coagulation factor levels [13–15]. For patients requiring long-term anticoagulation, VKA therapy should be stopped 4–5 days before surgery, and the INR should be measured before initiation of neuraxial block. For patients receiving a prophylactic dose of warfarin more than 24 h before surgery, INR measurements should be checked before neuraxial anesthesia. Neuraxial catheters can only be removed when the INR is less than 1.5 [13–15]. This value has been derived from studies that correlate hemostasis with clotting actor activity levels greater than 40 %.

Fondaparinux

Fondaparinux is approved since 2001, meanwhile with a broad spectrum of indications comparable to that of enoxaparin, including thromboembolic prophylaxis, treatment of venous thrombosis, pulmonary embolism, and unstable angina pectoris [30]. Fondaparinux was the first synthetic substance interfering with the factor Xa with some advantages over the LMWH (Tables 5.1 and 5.2). It further reduces the low molecular heparin structure to the essential pentasaccharide structure which is responsible for binding to antithrombin. The pentasaccharide binds like UFH and LMWH to antithrombin, producing a conformational change at the reactive site of antithrombin resulting in reversible binding to factor Xa with 700-fold higher affinity compared to heparins. This leads to a selective inhibition of factor Xa by mechanisms identical to LMWHs but without affecting the thrombin activity [22]. Only free factor Xa, but not factor Xa bound to the prothrombinase complex, is inhibited by fondaparinux [31]. Like all heparins, it is dependent on the presence and functionality of antithrombin. Fondaparinux catalyzes factor Xa inhibition by antithrombin but has no effect on the rate of thrombin inactivation. A meta-analysis by Turpie et al. showed that fondaparinux has greater efficacy in VTE prevention than LMWH [32]. Fondaparinux is eliminated via the renal route and is contraindicated in patients whose creatinine clearance is <30 ml/min. Fondaparinux is administered subcutaneously and has a longer half-life (14–21 h) than LMWHs allowing for single-daily dosing, with the first dose administered 6 h postoperatively [22] (Table 5.2). The risk of HIT is relatively low [33]. Fondaparinux does not require routine coagulation monitoring [34], except in patient with renal dysfunction [31, 35]. There are no clinically available reversal agents for fondaparinux, although partial reversal has recently been described with recombinant factor VIIa [33]. Fondaparinux is 100 % bioavailable and has a highly predictable pharmacokinetic profile.

The benefit-to-risk ratio of fondaparinux in preventing VTE was investigated in four randomized phase II trials in patients undergoing surgery for hip fracture, hip replacement, and major knee surgery. A meta-analysis of these trials demonstrated that fondaparinux reduced the incidence of venographically proven venous thromboembolism by 55.2 % compared with enoxaparin. The superior profile of fondaparinux over enoxaparin could also be demonstrated for proximal DVT with a reduction of 57.4 % [30]. Fondaparinux was also investigated for the initial treatment of venous thromboembolism in the MATISSE DVT trial [36] and the MATISSE PE [37] trials suggesting that fondaparinux is as effective and safe as UFH or LMWH for the initial treatment of patients with pulmonary embolism or deep vein thrombosis, respectively.

Fondaparinux and Neuraxial Anesthesia

Rosencher et al. recommend that fondaparinux to be started between 6 and 8 h after end of surgery [5]. Indwelling epidural catheters should not be removed until 36 h (or at least two half-lives) after the previous dose. The next dose should not be given until 12 h after catheter removal. The 48-h window required between two injections of fondaparinux is achieved by omitting one injection. In the EXPERT (*evaluation of Arixtra for the prevention of venous thromboembolism in daily practice*) study, this regimen was associated with safe catheter removal without affecting thromboprophylaxis efficacy. In patients receiving 2.5 mg fondaparinux daily for 3–5 weeks after major orthopedic surgery, the rate of symptomatic VTE was similar in patients with and without catheters. Moreover, no neuraxial hematoma was reported [38]. Although the risk of spinal hematoma is still unknown, spinal hematoma has been associated with the use of fondaparinux [13–15]. Therefore, close monitoring for clinical signs of neurological deterioration of patients receiving fondaparinux with neuraxial anesthesia and the need for postoperative indwelling epidural catheters are mandatory [5, 13–15].

Clinical Use of UFH, LMWH, Warfarin, and Fondaparinux

These anticoagulants have been successfully used in several clinical conditions caused by arterial and venous thromboembolism. The most important and clinically relevant are primary prophylaxis of VTE (DVT and PE) especially in high-risk orthopedic surgery patients and in different medical conditions, like the treatment and secondary prophylaxis of acute venous thromboembolism; prevention stroke in atrial fibrillation; and treatment of acute coronary syndromes [39].

UFH and LMWHs reduce venous thromboembolic complications by 60 % after hip and knee arthroplasties and in high-risk medical conditions including heart failure, prolonged immobilization in bed, etc. A further clinical field is their use in addition to dual antiplatelet therapy with aspirin and clopidogrel in acute coronary syndromes. Vitamin K antagonists reduce by >90 % the recurrence of venous thromboembolism and by 60 % cardioembolic stroke due to atrial fibrillation [24].

Fondaparinux is not only equally safe but also at least as effective as UFH and LMWH for the initial treatment of venous thromboembolism after once-daily subcutaneous injection [40, 41].

A limitation of UFH, LMWHs, and fondaparinux is the need of parenteral or subcutaneous administration which may complicate their use in the outpatient setting [22]. Oral VKA like warfarin and related compounds offers a clear advantage in the management of outpatients. On the other hand, they need regular laboratory monitoring with INR and frequent dosage tailoring due to many interactions with other drugs [24]. Despite the development of a standardized method to express the prothrombin time results (the international standardized ratio (INR)) with a substantial improvement in safety and efficacy, clinical use of vitamin K antagonists is still unsatisfactory mainly because many elderly patients do not have the autonomy to attend monitoring facilities at regular intervals.

The accuracy of UFH laboratory monitoring for the required dose adjustment is lagging behind that of VKA, as there is no result standardization obtained by different laboratory tests and reagents (activated clotting time, activated partial thromboplastin time). Therefore, the introduction of LMWHs, which only need dosage adjustment based upon patient weight in the absence of renal insufficiency, was a decisive step forward in patient management [42]. The introduction of fondaparinux was another improvement as this drug can be administered at a fixed dose of 2.5 mg sc without adjustment to body weight if patients have a renal function with a clearance <30 ml/min. Moreover, LMWHs and fondaparinux have significantly reduced the occurrence of nonanticoagulant side effects of UFH like thrombocytopenia and osteoporosis. Anyhow, a prudent use of these drugs is recommended, as there is always a potential risk because these drugs share the pentasaccharide structure with UFH [43].

For primary prophylaxis of VTE in high-risk orthopedic surgery, LMWHs are clearly more efficacious than UFH, but the incidence of venous thromboembolism remains however unacceptably high [44]. Subcutaneous fondaparinux in its recommended dose of 2.5 mg 6 h after surgery reduces venous thromboembolism by approximately 50 % compared with the LMWH enoxaparin. However, prolonged continuation of prophylaxis with LMWHs or fondaparinux for 30–40 days after discharge from hospital might be complicated if no nursing facilities are available for subcutaneous administration.

Most guidelines recommend 5–10 days of subcutaneous LMWHs for the treatment of acute venous thromboembolism [45]. The initial treatment with UFH, LMWHs, or fondaparinux is followed by bridging with vitamin K antagonists like warfarin. Warfarin is administrated for 3 months if venous thrombosis is provoked by transient risk factors (such as surgery, pregnancy, immobilization, etc.), for at least 6 months if thrombosis is spontaneous, and lifelong in the case of recurrent thrombosis [45, 46].

Actually, chronic atrial fibrillation represents the cardiological condition in which the use of anticoagulant therapy is definitely not satisfactory. In the population of over 60 years, 1 % develops this arrhythmia, with an increase to 10 % at the age of 80. Oral anticoagulant therapy with VKA is highly effective to reduce the rate of ischemic stroke by ≥60 %. In contrast, aspirin is three times less effective than vitamin K antagonists and offers no clear advantage concerning risk reduction of bleeding complications [47]. Unfortunately, adherence to guidelines is still very poor in most health care settings, although efficacy and cost effectiveness of anticoagulant prophylaxis have clearly been demonstrated [48]. It is obvious that there is a clear association between underuse of vitamin K antagonists and poorer outcome. The concern of physicians related to the high risk of bleeding in elderly patients and the poor patient compliance regarding regular drug intake and laboratory monitoring might be an explanation for this phenomenon [49].

Anticoagulants are also used for the treatment of cardiological atherothrombotic conditions like acute coronary syndromes, treated with or without vascular reperfusion techniques including pharmacological thrombolysis or percutaneous intervention. However, there is a need for improvement mainly due to the occurrence of bleeding complications in patients concomitantly treated with multiple drugs that impair hemostasis (UFH, LMWHs, or fondaparinux, administered on top of double or even triple antiplatelet agents like aspirin, ADP-receptor, and platelet glycoprotein IIb/IIIa inhibitors) [50]. To prevent reinfarction, traditional anticoagulants are the cornerstone of therapy. VKAs show high efficacy in this setting and are superior to monotherapy with aspirin [50]. However, they are rarely used by cardiologists due to the need for monitoring and the perceived high risk of bleeding. An oral drug with no need for monitoring would certainly positively influence cardiologists to prescribe anticoagulants for the prevention of secondary myocardial infarction, instead of the platelet function inhibitors currently prescribed [51].

All the above-mentioned limitations could be circumvented to some degree if new drugs with lower risk of bleeding and without the need of laboratory monitoring were available.

Conflicts of Interest None.

References

1. Hirsh J, Raschke R. Heparin and low-molecular-weight heparin: the seventh ACCP conference on antithrombotic and thrombolytic therapy. Chest. 2004;126(3 Suppl):188S–203.
2. Fareed J, Hoppensteadt DA, Fareed D, Demir M, Wahi R, Clarke M, et al. Survival of heparins, oral anticoagulants, and aspirin after the year 2010. Semin Thromb Hemost. 2008;34(1):58–73.
3. Harenberg J, Wehling M. Current and future prospects for anticoagulant therapy: inhibitors of factor Xa and factor IIa. Semin Thromb Hemost. 2008;34(1):39–57.
4. Mannucci PM, Poller L. Venous thrombosis and anticoagulant therapy. Br J Haematol. 2001;114(2):258–70.
5. Rosencher N, Bonnet MP, Sessler DI. Selected new antithrombotic agents and neuraxial anaesthesia for major orthopaedic surgery: management strategies. Anaesthesia. 2007;62(11): 1154–60.
6. Geerts WH. Prevention of venous thromboembolism in high-risk patients. Hematology Am Soc Hematol Educ Program. 2006:462–6.
7. Kurmis AP. Review article: thromboprophylaxis after total hip replacement. J Orthop Surg (Hong Kong). 2010;18(1):92–7.
8. Choi BY, Huo MH. Venous thromboembolism following total knee replacement. J Surg Orthop Adv. 2007;16(1):31–5.
9. Rogers BA, Little NJ. Thromboprophylaxis in orthopaedic surgery: a clinical review. J Perioper Pract. 2010;20(10):358–62.
10. Abad Rico JI, Llau Pitarch JV, Rocha E. Overview of venous thromboembolism. Drugs. 2010;70 Suppl 2:3–10.
11. Duggan ST, Scott LJ, Plosker GL. Rivaroxaban: a review of its use for the prevention of venous thromboembolism after total hip or knee replacement surgery. Drugs. 2009;69(13):1829–51.
12. Bergqvist D. Review of fondaparinux sodium injection for the prevention of venous thromboembolism in patients undergoing surgery. Vasc Health Risk Manag. 2006;2(4):365–70.
13. Horlocker TT, Wedel DJ, Benzon H, Brown DL, Enneking FK, Heit JA, et al. Regional anesthesia in the anticoagulated patient: defining the risks (the second ASRA consensus conference on neuraxial anesthesia and anticoagulation). Reg Anesth Pain Med. 2003;28(3):172–97.
14. Horlocker TT, Wedel DJ, Rowlingson JC, Enneking FK. Executive summary: regional anesthesia in the patient receiving antithrombotic or thrombolytic therapy: American Society of regional anesthesia and pain medicine evidence-based guidelines (third edition). Reg Anesth Pain Med. 2010;35(1):102–5.
15. Horlocker TT, Wedel DJ, Rowlingson JC, Enneking FK, Kopp SL, Benzon HT, et al. Regional anesthesia in the patient receiving antithrombotic or thrombolytic therapy: American Society of regional anesthesia and pain medicine evidence-based guidelines (third edition). Reg Anesth Pain Med. 2010;35(1):64–101.
16. Gogarten W. The influence of new antithrombotic drugs on regional anesthesia. Curr Opin Anaesthesiol. 2006;19(5):545–50.
17. Haas S, Schellong S. New anticoagulants: from bench to bedside. Hamostaseologie. 2007;27(1):41–7.
18. Harbrecht U. Old and new anticoagulants. Hamostaseologie. 2011;31(1):21–7.
19. Levy JH, Key NS, Azran MS. Novel oral anticoagulants: implications in the perioperative setting. Anesthesiology. 2010;113(3):726–45.
20. Hong MS, Amanullah AM. Heparin-induced thrombocytopenia: a practical review. Rev Cardiovasc Med. 2010;11(1):13–25.
21. Kozek-Langenecker SA. Perioperative coagulation monitoring. Best Pract Res Clin Anaesthesiol. 2010;24(1):27–40.

22. Hirsh J, Bauer KA, Donati MB, Gould M, Samama MM, Weitz JI. Parenteral anticoagulants: American College of chest physicians evidence-based clinical practice guidelines (8th edition). Chest. 2008;133(6 Suppl):141S–59.
23. Weitz JI. Low-molecular-weight heparins. N Engl J Med. 1997;337(10):688–98.
24. Ansell J, Hirsh J, Hylek E, Jacobson A, Crowther M, Palareti G. Pharmacology and management of the vitamin K antagonists: American College of chest physicians evidence-based clinical practice guidelines (8th edition). Chest. 2008;133(6 Suppl):160S–98.
25. Hart RG, Benavente O, McBride R, Pearce LA. Antithrombotic therapy to prevent stroke in patients with atrial fibrillation: a meta-analysis. Ann Intern Med. 1999;131(7):492–501.
26. Haas S. Medical indications and considerations for future clinical decision making. Thromb Res. 2003;109 Suppl 1:S31–7.
27. Eriksson BI, Quinlan DJ. Oral anticoagulants in development: focus on thromboprophylaxis in patients undergoing orthopaedic surgery. Drugs. 2006;66(11):1411–29.
28. Levy JH, Tanaka KA, Dietrich W. Perioperative hemostatic management of patients treated with vitamin K antagonists. Anesthesiology. 2008;109(5):918–26.
29. West KL, Adamson C, Hoffman M. Prophylactic correction of the international normalized ratio in neurosurgery: a brief review of a brief literature. J Neurosurg. 2011;114(1):9–18.
30. Turpie AG, Bauer KA, Eriksson BI, Lassen MR. Fondaparinux vs enoxaparin for the prevention of venous thromboembolism in major orthopedic surgery: a meta-analysis of 4 randomized double-blind studies. Arch Intern Med. 2002;162(16):1833–40.
31. Blick SK, Orman JS, Wagstaff AJ, Scott LJ. Fondaparinux sodium: a review of its use in the management of acute coronary syndromes. Am J Cardiovasc Drugs. 2008;8(2):113–25.
32. Turpie AG, Eriksson BI, Lassen MR, Bauer KA. A meta-analysis of fondaparinux versus enoxaparin in the prevention of venous thromboembolism after major orthopaedic surgery. J South Orthop Assoc. 2002;11(4):182–8.
33. Lisman T, Bijsterveld NR, Adelmeijer J, Meijers JC, Levi M, Nieuwenhuis HK, et al. Recombinant factor VIIa reverses the in vitro and ex vivo anticoagulant and profibrinolytic effects of fondaparinux. J Thromb Haemost. 2003;1(11):2368–73.
34. Giangrande PL. Fondaparinux (arixtra): a new anticoagulant. Int J Clin Pract. 2002;56(8):615–7.
35. Bauer KA. Fondaparinux sodium: a selective inhibitor of factor Xa. Am J Health Syst Pharm. 2001;58 Suppl 2:S14–7.
36. Buller HR, Davidson BL, Decousus H, Gallus A, Gent M, Piovella F, et al. Fondaparinux or enoxaparin for the initial treatment of symptomatic deep venous thrombosis: a randomized trial. Ann Intern Med. 2004;140(11):867–73.
37. Buller HR, Davidson BL, Decousus H, Gallus A, Gent M, Piovella F, et al. Subcutaneous fondaparinux versus intravenous unfractionated heparin in the initial treatment of pulmonary embolism. N Engl J Med. 2003;349(18):1695–702.
38. Singelyn FJ, Verheyen CC, Piovella F, Van Aken HK, Rosencher N. The safety and efficacy of extended thromboprophylaxis with fondaparinux after major orthopedic surgery of the lower limb with or without a neuraxial or deep peripheral nerve catheter: the EXPERT Study. Anesth Analg. 2007;105(6):1540–7. table of contents.
39. Bates SM, Weitz JI. New anticoagulants: beyond heparin, low-molecular-weight heparin and warfarin. Br J Pharmacol. 2005;144(8):1017–28.
40. Petitou M, Duchaussoy P, Herbert JM, Duc G, El Hajji M, Branellec JF, et al. The synthetic pentasaccharide fondaparinux: first in the class of antithrombotic agents that selectively inhibit coagulation factor Xa. Semin Thromb Hemost. 2002;28(4):393–402.
41. Bauer KA, Hawkins DW, Peters PC, Petitou M, Herbert JM, van Boeckel CA, et al. Fondaparinux, a synthetic pentasaccharide: the first in a new class of antithrombotic agents the selective factor Xa inhibitors. Cardiovasc Drug Rev. 2002;20(1):37–52.
42. Hirsh J, O'Donnell M, Eikelboom JW. Beyond unfractionated heparin and warfarin: current and future advances. Circulation. 2007;116(5):552–60.

43. Warkentin TE, Greinacher A. Heparin-induced thrombocytopenia: recognition, treatment, and prevention: the seventh ACCP conference on antithrombotic and thrombolytic therapy. Chest. 2004;126(3 Suppl):311S–37.
44. Geerts WH, Pineo GF, Heit JA, Bergqvist D, Lassen MR, Colwell CW, et al. Prevention of venous thromboembolism: the seventh ACCP conference on antithrombotic and thrombolytic therapy. Chest. 2004;126(3 Suppl):338S–400.
45. Buller HR, Agnelli G, Hull RD, Hyers TM, Prins MH, Raskob GE. Antithrombotic therapy for venous thromboembolic disease: the seventh ACCP conference on antithrombotic and thrombolytic therapy. Chest. 2004;126(3 Suppl):401S–28.
46. Agrawal YK, Vaidya H, Bhatt H, Manna K, Brahmkshatriya P. Recent advances in the treatment of thromboembolic diseases: venous thromboembolism. Med Res Rev. 2007;27(6): 891–914.
47. Singer DE, Albers GW, Dalen JE, Go AS, Halperin JL, Manning WJ. Antithrombotic therapy in atrial fibrillation: the seventh ACCP conference on antithrombotic and thrombolytic therapy. Chest. 2004;126(3 Suppl):429S–56.
48. Marcucci M, Iorio A, Nobili A, Tettamanti M, Pasina L, Marengoni A, et al. Factors affecting adherence to guidelines for antithrombotic therapy in elderly patients with atrial fibrillation admitted to internal medicine wards. Eur J Intern Med. 2010;21(6):516–23.
49. Braun S, Voller H, Soppa C, Taborski U. Update of guidelines for patient self-management of oral anticoagulation. Dtsch Med Wochenschr. 2009;134(14):695–700.
50. Harrington RA, Becker RC, Ezekowitz M, Meade TW, O'Connor CM, Vorchheimer DA, et al. Antithrombotic therapy for coronary artery disease: the seventh ACCP conference on antithrombotic and thrombolytic therapy. Chest. 2004;126(3 Suppl):513S–48.
51. Menon V, Harrington RA, Hochman JS, Cannon CP, Goodman SD, Wilcox RG, et al. Thrombolysis and adjunctive therapy in acute myocardial infarction: the seventh ACCP conference on antithrombotic and thrombolytic therapy. Chest. 2004;126(3 Suppl):549S–75.

Chapter 6
New Drugs for Thromboprophylaxis: Apixaban, Dabigatran, Rivaroxaban

Raquel Ferrandis

Abstract Recently, new direct oral anticoagulant agents have been developed, and some of them have received approval for thromboprophylaxis after hip or knee arthroplasty, with other medical and surgical indications being accepted or investigated in several ongoing studies. The most developed ones are apixaban, rivaroxaban, and dabigatran. This chapter provides a review of their pharmacology and a temporary update of their indications, giving the basis for their management in orthopedic surgery.

Keywords Anticoagulant • Apixaban • Rivaroxaban • Dabigatran Thromboprophylaxis • Orthopedic surgery • Regional anesthesia

Introduction: Are New Drugs for Thromboprophylaxis Necessary?

Traditional methods of anticoagulation and thromboprophylaxis have involved vitamin K antagonists (VKA) (such as warfarin or acenocumarol), heparin (both low molecular weight, LMWH, and unfractionated, UFH), fondaparinux, and antiplatelet agents. Between them, the ACCP guidelines recommend in total hip (THR) and knee (TKR) replacement prophylaxis with LMWH, VKA, or fondaparinux for all patient groups (grade 1A) and against aspirin alone (grade 1A) and low-dose UFH alone (grade 1A) [1].

R. Ferrandis, M.D., Ph.D.
Department of Anaesthesiology and Critical Care,
Hospital Clinic Universitari de València,
Avda Blasco Ibáñez 17, 46006 Valencia, Spain

Human Physiology Department,
School of Medicine, Valencia University, Valencia, Spain
e-mail: raquelferrandis@gmail.com

J.V. Llau (ed.), *Thromboembolism in Orthopedic Surgery*,
DOI 10.1007/978-1-4471-4336-9_6, © Springer-Verlag London 2013

But current anticoagulant drugs, despite their proven efficacy, have significant limitations that have prompted the development of new agents with more efficacy and a better safety profile [2, 3]. We can mention, for example, the low predictable response to VKA and their high potential for drug–drug interactions or the need of parenteral administration of heparin. New drugs have focused their development on the characteristics of the ideal anticoagulant that have been described as follows [4]:

- Possibility of oral (one tablet, once daily) and parenteral (once daily) administration
- High effectivity in reducing thromboembolic events
- Low rate of complications (focus on bleeding)
- Possibility of reversal if necessary (specific antidote)
- Predictable pharmacokinetics, predictable dose response
- Rapid onset of action
- No need for routine monitoring or platelet count
- Wide therapeutic window
- No dose adjustment required
- No interaction with other drugs
- Low nonspecific plasma protein binding
- Inhibition of both free and clot-bound activated coagulation factors

Recently, new direct oral anticoagulant agents have been developed, and some of them have received approval for thromboprophylaxis after hip or knee arthroplasty, with other medical and surgical indications being accepted or investigated in several ongoing studies. Many reviews have been made during the last years about these drugs, some of highly recommended lecture [5–7]. In this chapter, we will update the management of the most developed ones, apixaban, dabigatran and rivaroxaban, mainly in thromboprophylaxis of total hip and knee arthroplasty.

Apixaban

Apixaban (Eliquis®, Bristol-Myers Squibb/Pfizer EEIG, United Kingdom) is an orally bioavailable, highly selective, reversible, and direct acting factor Xa inhibitor. After oral intake, apixaban has more than 50 % bioavailability and reaches peak plasma concentration in 30 min to 4 h, with a terminal half-life round 12 h. The drug is absorbed in the gastrointestinal tract. It is metabolized in the liver by cytochrome (CYP3A4)-dependent and cytochrome-independent mechanisms, and it is eliminated through both the renal (30 %) and the fecal routes (70 %) [8]. The results of in vitro studies suggest that the metabolic drug–drug interaction potential is low; also food does not interfere with apixaban absorption [9]. The most important pharmacology characteristics are summed up in Table 6.1 [10].

Because there is limited clinical data, apixaban is not recommended in patients with creatinine clearance <15 ml/min, in patients undergoing dialysis, or in patients with severe hepatic impairment, and it is to be used with caution in patients with severe renal impairment (creatine clearance 15–29 ml/min) and in patients with

Table 6.1 Pharmacokinetic properties of new anticoagulants

	Apixaban	Dabigatran	Rivaroxaban
Mechanism of action	Direct Xa inhibitor	Direct IIa inhibitor	Direct Xa inhibitor
Protein binding (%)	35	>90	40–59
Substrate of transporters (P-gp)	Yes	Yes	Yes
Half-life (h)	8–15	14–17	5–9
Substrate or CYP enzymes	Minor (CYP3A4)	No	Major (CYP3A4, CYP2J2)
Elimination	70 % unchanged 30 % inactive metabolism	100 % unchanged drug + active metabolism	50 % unchanged 50 % inactive metabolism
Route of elimination	25 % urine 70 % feces	80 % urine 20 % feces	70 % urine 30 % feces

Table 6.2 Apixaban for thromboprophylaxis in orthopedic surgery

	ADVANCE-2		ADVANCE-3	
Setting	TKR		THR	
No. of patients	1,528	1,529	2,708	2,699
Drug	Apixaban	Enoxaparin	Apixaban	Enoxaparin
Dose	2.5 mg BD	40 mg OD	2.5 mg BD	40 mg OD
First dose	12–24 h postop	12 h preop	12–24 h postop	12 h preop
Treatment duration (day)	10–14	10–14	35	35
Total VTE/all cause of death (%)	15.06[a]	24.37	1.4[a]	3.9
Major VTE (%)	1.09[a]	2.17	0.5[a]	1.1
Major bleeding (%)	0.6	0.9	0.8	0.7
Clinically relevant bleeding (%)	2.9	3.8	4.1	4.5

VTE venous thromboembolism, *TKR* total knee replacement, *THR* total hip replacement, *BD* twice daily, *OD* once daily, *preop* preoperative, *postop* postoperative
[a]Clinical significant

mild to moderate hepatic impairment (Child Plugh A or B). No dose adjustment is required in these patients. No dose adjustment is either required because of body weight, gender, or elderly. The use of apixaban is also not recommended in patients receiving concomitant systemic treatment with strong inhibitors of both CYP3A4 and P-gp inducers, such as azole antimycotics and HIV-protease inhibitors [10].

As other new anticoagulants the first studies have been rolled in thromboprophylaxis after orthopedic surgery (Table 6.2). In ADVANCE-1 [11], investigators compared apixaban 2.5 mg twice daily, starting 12–24 h after knee replacement, with postoperative enoxaparin 30 mg twice daily, but the study did not meet statistical criteria for non-inferiority, although reduced bleeding was reported with apixaban. Then, in ADVANCE-2 [12], apixaban 2.5 mg twice daily has been compared with the widely use regimen of enoxaparin 40 mg/day; it showed that apixaban was more effective for prevention of VTE, without increasing bleeding risk. ADVANCE-3 [13], conducted in patients undergoing hip replacement, showed that thromboprophylaxis with apixaban (2.5 mg twice daily), as compared with enoxaparin (40 mg/day), was associated with lower rate of venous thromboembolism, without increasing bleeding. Based on these studies, apixaban has recently been approved by the EMA (EMA240842/2011) to prevent venous thromboembolic events in adults following hip or knee replacement operation.

About clinical studies, in AVERROES, apixaban 5 mg twice daily, versus acetylsalicylic acid, reduced the risk of stroke or systemic embolism without significantly increasing the risk of major bleeding or intracranial hemorrhage in atrial fibrillation patients who have failed or are unsuitable for vitamin K antagonist treatment [14]. The phase 3 study APPRAISE 2 observed a dose-related increase in bleeding more pronounced than the reduction in ischemic events with the addition of apixaban to antiplatelet therapy in patients with recent acute coronary syndrome [15]. Nowadays, other studies are being conducted: ARISTOTLE, a study to compare apixaban and warfarin in atrial fibrillation patients [16]; AMPLIFY that will compare apixaban (10 mg twice daily for 7 days, followed by apixaban 5 mg, twice daily for 6 months) to a standard strategy using enoxaparin followed by VKA in patients with acute VTE; and ADOPT that compares apixaban with enoxaparin for the prevention of VTE in hospitalized medically ill patients (NCT00457002).

Dabigatran

Dabigatran (Pradaxa®, Boehringer Ingelheim International GmbH, Germany) is a direct thrombin inhibitor. It is the unique oral agent of this class, and there are three intravenous agents currently available (lepirudin, bivalirudin, and argatroban) [17]. Dabigatran etexilate is a prodrug that is converted to dabigatran, the active molecule, by esterases. Peak dabigatran plasma concentration occurs 30–120 min after oral administration, with a bioavailability of 5–6 %. Because its absorption requires an acidic environment, the oral capsule contains tartaric acid, and it must not be manipulated, it should be swallowed as a whole with water, with or without food. The dabigatran half-life extends to 8 h after a single-dose administration and up to 17 h after multiple doses. As much as 80 % of the drug is excreted unchanged by the kidneys and 20 % by the biliary system after being conjugated (see Table 6.1). Therefore, the drug is contraindicated in patients with creatine clearance less than 30 ml/min, and it is not recommended in patients with elevated liver enzymes more than two times the upper limit of normal [18, 19].

Although drug interactions with new anticoagulants must be viewed with caution, as we will know more as their use becomes more wide spread in clinical practice, there are some points to bear in mind. Dabigatran is a substrate for the P-glycoprotein transport system, and then, it is not recommended in patients treated with quinidine, a potent P-glycoprotein inducer. But the interaction with other P-glycoprotein substrates is not clinically relevant, such as atorvastatin [20] or digoxin [21]. Not relevant is the interaction of dabigatran and ranitidine and other proton pump inhibitors [22].

Table 6.3 Dabigatran for thromboprophylaxis in orthopedic surgery

	RE-NOVATE		RE-MODEL		RE-MOBILIZE	
Setting	THR		TKR		TKR	
No. of patients	1,163–1,146	1,154	703–679	694	871–857	868
Drug	Dabigatran	Enoxaparin	Dabigatran	Enoxaparin	Dabigatran	Enoxaparin
Dose	150–220	40 mg od	150–220	40 mg od	150–220	30 mg bid
First dose	1–4 h postop	12 h preop	1–4 h postop	12 h preop	6–12 h postop	12 h postop
Treatment duration (day)	28–35	28–35	6–10	6–10	12–15	12–15
Total VTE/all cause of death (%)	8.6–6	6.7	40.5–36.4	37.7	33.7–31.1	25.3
Major bleeding (%)	1.3–3	1.6	1.3–1.5	1.3	0.6–0.6	1.4
Clinically relevant bleeding (%)	4.7–4.2	3.5	6.8–5.9	5.3	2.5–2.7	2.4

VTE venous thromboembolism, *TKR* total knee replacement, *THR* total hip replacement, *bid* twice daily, *od* once daily, *preop* preoperative, *postop* postoperative

Based on the studies RE-NOVATE [23], in patients undergoing THR, and RE-MOBILIZE [24] and RE-MODEL [25], in patients undergoing TKR, dabigatran etexilate has been already licensed for the thromboprophylaxis in THR and TKR surgery, with an accepted dose of 220 mg once daily (Table 6.3). The dose has to be adjusted to half dose (150 mg daily) in patients with moderate renal insufficiency (creatinine clearance between 30 and 50 ml/min), elderly (aged 75 or more), and patients on amiodarone treatment. The first dose is given orally in the postoperative period, between 1 and 4 h after the end of surgery, as a half dose (110 or 75 mg) [22].

Dabigatran was studied in a non-inferiority trial in patients with acute venous thromboembolism (VTE) (RE-COVER) [26]. After the initial anticoagulation with heparin, the study compared oral dabigatran 150 mg twice daily with warfarin adjusted to achieve an INR 2–3. Dabigatran was as effective as warfarin, with a similar safety profile, and it did not require laboratory monitoring. A second VTE treatment study has recently been completed (RE-COVER II, NCT00680186). Moreover, two trials have been conducted for the secondary prevention of VTE for 3–6 months (RE-MEDY, NCT00329238) or 6–18 months (RE-SONATE NCT00558259).

The RE-LY study evaluated the efficacy and safety of two doses of dabigatran (150 and 110 mg, both given twice daily) relative to warfarin in patients with atrial fibrillation [27]. The study concluded that dabigatran at a dose of 110 mg was associated with rates of stroke and systemic embolism similar to warfarin and lower rates of major hemorrhage. The dose of 150 mg was associated with lower rates of stroke and systemic embolism but similar rates of hemorrhage. As a result of these data, the FDA has approved dabigatran 150 mg twice daily for stroke prevention in atrial fibrillation. Furthermore, a report of the American College of Cardiology Foundation/American Heart Association Task Force on practice guidelines has recently given a class I/level of evidence B recommendation [28]. Also on April 2011, the Committee for Medicinal Products for Human Use (CHMP) of EMA adopted a positive opinion about the indication of Pradaxa for prevention of stroke and systemic embolism in adults with nonvalvular atrial fibrillation with one or more risk factors. In patients with atrial fibrillation, who completed the RE-LY trial, a long-term safety study is ongoing, RELY-ABLE (NCT00808067).

For secondary prevention after an acute coronary syndrome, the RE-DEEM trial (phase II) revealed that dabigatran, in addition to dual antiplatelet therapy, was associated with a dose-dependent increase in bleeding events and significantly reduced coagulation activity [29]. Although the total number of patients suffering ischemic cardiovascular events during the study was low, with minor differences between the treatment groups, the net clinical benefit of dabigatran needs to be evaluated in a phase III study.

Rivaroxaban

Rivaroxaban (Xarelto®, Bayer HealthCare AG, Germany) is an oral direct FXa inhibitor. It has predictable pharmacokinetics with high oral bioavailability (about 80 %) and a rapid onset of action. The peak level is reached at 2–4 h, being slightly enhanced by food intake. Its half-life is 5–9 h. Approximately 66 % of the administered dose undergoes metabolic degradation, with half then being eliminated by renal clearance and the other half through the fecal route. The final 33 % of the administered dose undergoes direct renal excretion as unchanged active substance in the urine, mainly through active renal secretion (see Table 6.1) [9, 30].

The first indication approved for rivaroxaban was thromboprophylaxis in patients undergoing hip or knee arthroplasty, after the four studies RECORD, RECORD 1 and 2 in THR, and RECORD 3 and 4 in TKR (Table 6.4) [31–34]. The recommended dose is 10 mg daily, starting 6–8 h after wound closure. It is not necessary to adjust the dose in the presence of mild or severe renal impairment (creatinine clearance 15–80 ml/min). Rivaroxaban is contraindicated in hepatic disease with coagulopathy and clinical bleeding risk, and it should be used with caution in cases of moderate hepatic impairment (Child Pugh B).

About drug interactions, with the above cautions mentioned, rivaroxaban is not recommended in patients treated with potent inhibitors of CYP3A4 and P-gp, as azole antimycotics or systemic HIV-protease inhibitors [35]. Not of clinical significance was the interaction with moderate inhibitors such as clarithromycin, erythromycin, or rifampicin [35]. Other substrates of CYP3A4 and P-gp, as midazolam, digoxina, or atorvastatin, given with rivaroxaban showed no clinically significant

Table 6.4 Rivaroxaban for thromboprophylaxis in orthopedic surgery

Setting	RECORD 1		RECORD 2		RECORD 3		RECORD 4	
	THR	THR	THR	THR	TKR	TKR	TKR	TKR
No. of patients	2,209	2,224	1,228	1,229	1,220	1,239	1,526	1,508
Drug	Rivaroxaban	Enoxaparin	Rivaroxaban	Enoxaparin	Rivaroxaban	Enoxaparin	Rivaroxaban	Enoxaparin
Dose	10 mg OD	40 mg OD	10 mg OD	40 mg OD	10 mg OD	40 mg OD	10 mg OD	30 mg BD
First dose	6–8 h postop	12 h preop	6–8 h postop	12 h preop	6–8 h postop	12 h preop	6–8 h postop	12–24 h postop
Treatment duration (day)	30–40	30–40	30–40	14	14	14	14	14
Total VTE/all cause of death (%)	1.1[a]	3.7	2.0[a]	9.3	9.6[a]	18.9	6.9[a]	10.1
Major VTE (%)	0.2[a]	2	0.6[a]	5.1	1[a]	2.6	1.2	2
Major Bleeding (%)	0.3	0.1	0.1	0.1	0.6	0.5	0.7	0.3
Clinically relevant bleeding (%)	2.9	2.4	3.3	2.7	2.7	2.3	2.6	2

VTE venous thromboembolism, *TKR* total knee replacement, *THR* total hip replacement, *BD* twice daily, *OD* once daily, *preop* preoperative, *postop* postoperative

[a]Clinical significant

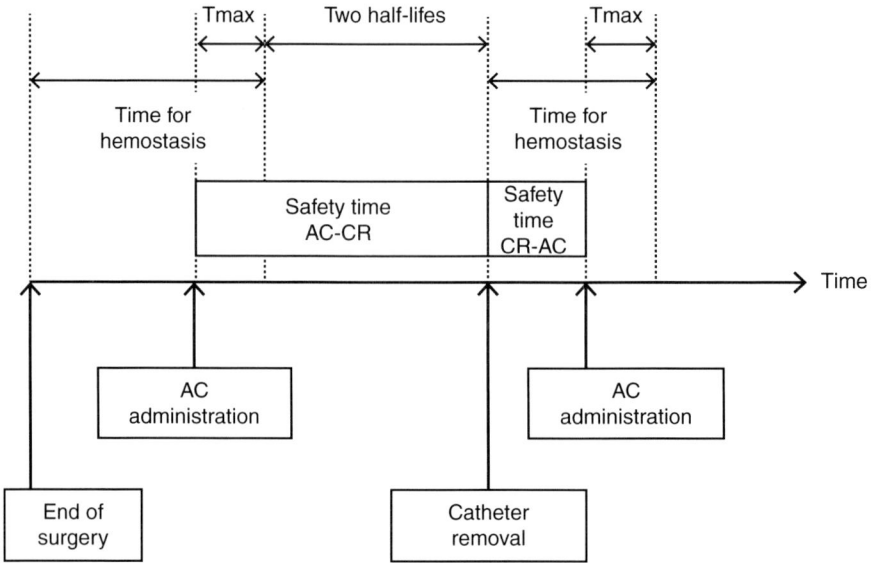

Fig. 6.1 Recommendations for the managing of the catheter based on pharmacokinetics of antico-agulant (see text). T_{max} Time to peak plasma level, *AC-CR* Safety time between anticoagulant dose and catheter removal, *CR-AC* Safety time between catheter removal and next anticoagulant dose (Modified from Llau and Ferrandis [5]. With permission from Wolters Kluwer Health)

interactions [35]. No effect in bioavailability and pharmacokinetic was noted when rivaroxaban was coadministered with antiacids and H_2 receptor antagonists [36].

Rivaroxaban (15 mg twice daily for 3 weeks, followed by 20 mg once daily) was evaluated for the treatment of acute symptomatic deep vein thrombosis (EINSTEIN-DVT) [37]. The study showed that rivaroxaban alone is as effective as standard therapy (enoxaparin followed by VKA), with similar safety. After these results, on September 2011, the Committee for Medicinal Products for Human Use (CHMP) of EMA has adopted a positive opinion about this indication. When treatment is continued (EINSTEIN-Extension) (rivaroxaban 20 mg once daily for an additional 6–12 months), rivaroxaban is effective in preventing recurrences and has an acceptable risk of bleeding [37]. A study for the treatment of pulmonary embolism (EINSTEIN-PE, NCT00438777) is ongoing.

The ROCKET-AF trial suggest, based on preliminary results, the efficacy and safety of rivaroxaban (20 mg once daily) as an alternative to warfarin for the prevention of thromboembolism in high-risk patients with atrial fibrillation [38], together with the acute treatment of VTE, the EMA adopted appositive opinion about this indication on September 2011.

In ATLAS-ACS 1 (phase II), a trial of patients with recent acute coronary syndrome, rivaroxaban increased the risk of clinically significant bleeding in a dose-dependent manner when compare to placebo, while leading to a nonsignificant reduction in the primary composite efficacy endpoint. As a result, a phase III trial (ATLAS-ACS 2; NCT00809965) is comparing two doses of rivaroxaban, 2.5 and 5 mg twice daily.

Table 6.5 Recommendations for anticoagulant agents related to the practice of regional anesthesia

	Half-life (h)	Time of peak level (h)	Safety time RA-AC (h)	Safety time AC-RC (h)	Safety time CR-AC (h)
LMWH	4–6	3–4	4–6	10–12	4–6
Fondaparinux	17–21	1–2	6	36	12
Apixaban	8–15	3	6	20–30	6
Dabigatran	14–17	2–4	2–4	NR	2–4
Rivaroxaban	5–9	2.5–4	4–6	18	6

RA-AC interval of time between the performance of the regional anesthetic technique and the administration of the next anticoagulant dose, *AC-RC* interval of time between the administration of the last anticoagulant dose and the removal of the catheter, *CR-AC* interval of time between the removal of the catheter and the administration of the next anticoagulant dose, *NR* not recommended

New Oral Anticoagulants and Regional Anesthesia

The performance of regional anesthesia in patients receiving anticoagulant drugs must be managed taking into account the type of anesthetic–analgesic technique to be carried out, the characteristics of the anticoagulant, the procedure-related risk factors, and additional personal risk factors [39–41]. Recently, Rosencher et al. [40] propose that safety time intervals should be based on the pharmacological profile (pharmacokinetics and pharmacodynamics) of each specific drug, mainly the time required to reach maximal concentration, the half-life, and the dose regimen. The rules based on the pharmacokinetics can be summarized as follows (Fig. 6.1):

1. The first dose of the anticoagulant after a neuraxial puncture must be administered so as to ensure an interval of at least 8 h between the end of surgery and the peak plasma level of the drug.
2. The removal of a deep catheter must be delayed at least two half-lives of the anticoagulant following the last peak plasma level (when there is only 25 % of the circulating drug remaining).
3. The safety interval between the removal of the catheter and the next anticoagulant administration must be delayed by a period calculated from the hemostasis time minus the peak plasma level of the drug (the longer the peak level, the shorter the time delays).

Based on the above pharmacokinetics, a summary of the main recommendations for current and new anticoagulants is shown in Table 6.5. About new anticoagulants:

Spinal Anesthesia

After performing spinal atraumatic anesthesia, the first dose of dabigatran etexilate can be administrated at 1–4 h after the end of surgery, 4–6 h for ribaroxaban, and 6 h for apixaban. But, if a traumatic/hemorrhagic puncture occurs, the first dose of any anticoagulant should be delayed for 24 h.

Epidural Anesthesia

Dabigatran etexilate cannot be administrated if epidural anesthesia with the insertion of a permanent catheter for postoperative analgesia has been performed. Talking about rivaroxaban, the first dose, with the catheter in place, will be administered at 6–10 h after the end of surgery. Between the administration of the drug and the removal of the catheter, it is necessary to wait for an interval of at least 18 h, being recommendable to prolong this safety window until 22–26 h if the patient is elderly, because of the prolonged half-life in this case. The minimal interval between catheter removal and next dose of rivaroxaban should be 6 h.

There is no clinical experience with the use of apixaban with indwelling intrathecal or epidural catheters, but based on the pharmacokinetics, a time interval of 20–30 h between the last dose of apixaban and the catheter withdrawal should elapse (i.e., at least one dose should be omitted). The next dose may be given at least 6 h after the removal.

Although there is few data available, switching from parenteral anticoagulants treatment to dabigatran, rivaroxaban, or apixaban, the oral anticoagulant is not recommended to start before the next scheduled dose of the parenteral anticoagulant would have been due.

Continuous Peripheral Nerve Blocks (CPNB)

Upon performing CPNB, bleeding complications are usually less important than those associated with neuraxial blocks. But, an eventual bleed derived from a CPNB can lead to a mechanical compression of the nerve with nerve palsy and could even lead to life-threatening bleeding [25] if undiagnosed. Recently, ultrasound-guided peripheral nerve blockade has become a valuable tool; nevertheless, it cannot be assumed in clinical practice as the new gold standard for peripheral regional anesthesia in absolute terms of efficacy and safety.

The proposal for the practice of CPNB by the ASA [26] states that peripheral nerve blocks must have the same safety profile as neuraxial blocks. Although it may be too stringent to all peripheral nerve blocks, it seems necessary to maintain caution at least in some kind of blocks (mainly performed in a noncompressible area: posterior lumbar plexus, sciatic parasacral, or infraclavicular blocks) so as to emulate the safety profile of neuraxial blocks.

Conclusions

New drugs for thromboprophylaxis are each day less future and more present. The new oral anticoagulants that have all began as thromboprophylaxis in orthopedic surgery, offering an alternative to parenteral heparins, are nowadays widespread in medical settings. This chapter must be considered a review of the pharmacology of these drugs and a temporary update of their indications.

As new drugs, great care should be taken in the management of new direct oral anticoagulants, in a special way in patients with hepatic or renal impairment, with concomitant drugs or with indwelling epidural catheters. In this setting, this chapter (together with the one about bridge therapy) tries to give the basis, but new indications are being approved, more patients and more type of patients are been included, and different dosage are being studied, so the scenario is changing and will be changing the next years.

Maybe, the most important point will be to keep in mind the pharmacokinetic basis. In fact, the different guides and recommendations are based on pharmacokinetics to propose the time intervals. Nevertheless, as there is no experience, the clinician should be cautious till the time and the experience tell us the correct way to go.

References

1. Geerts WH, Bergqvist D, Pineo GF, Heilt JA, Samama CM, Lassen MR, et al. Prevention of venous thromboembolism: American College of Chest Physicians evidence-based clinical practice guideline (8th edition). Chest. 2008;133:381S–435.
2. Weitz JI, Hirsh J, Samama MM. New antithrombotic drugs. Chest. 2008;133:234S–56.
3. Hirsh J, O'Donnell M, Weitz JI. New anticoagulants. Blood. 2005;105:453–63.
4. Bounameaux H. The novel anticoagulants: entering a new era. Swiss Med Wkly. 2009; 139:60–4.
5. Llau JV, Ferrandis R. New anticoagulants and regional anesthesia. Curr Opin Anaesthesiol. 2009;22(5):661–6.
6. Garcia D, Libby E, Crowther MA. The new oral anticoagulants. Blood. 2010;115:15–20.
7. Galanis T, Thomson L, Palladino M, Merli GJ. New oral anticoagulants. J Thromb Thrombolysis. 2011;31:310–20.
8. Raghavan N, Frost CE, Yu Z, He K, Zhang H, Humpreys WG. Apixaban metabolism and pharmacokinetics after oral administration to humans. Drug Metab Dispos. 2009;37(1): 74–81.
9. Eriksson BI, Quinlan DJ, Weitz JI. Comparative pharmacodynamics and pharmacokinetics of oral direct thrombin and factor Xa inhibitors development. Clin Pharmacokinet. 2009;48: 1–22.
10. Eliquis (apixaban). Summary of product characteristics, Bristol Myers Squibb/Pfizer EEIG. http://ec.europa.eu/health/documments/community-register/2011/20110518102349/anx_102349-en.pdf. (Accessed March 30th 2012)
11. Lassen MR, Raskob GE, Gallus A, Pineo G, Chen D, Portman RJ. Apixaban or enoxaparin for thromboprophylaxis after knee replacement. N Engl J Med. 2009;361:594–604.
12. Lassen MR, Raskob GE, Galus A, Pineo G, Chen D, Hornick P, the ADVANCE-2 Investigators. Apixaban versus enoxaparin for thromboprophylaxis after knee replacement (ADVANCE-2): a randomized double-blind trial. Lancet. 2010;375:807–15.
13. Lassen MR, Gallus A, Raskob GE, Pineo G, Chen D, Ramirez LM, the ADVANCE-3 Investigators. Apixaban versus enoxaparin for thromboprophylaxis after hip replacement. N Engl J Med. 2010;363:2487–98.
14. Connolly SJ, Eikelboom J, Joyner C, Diener HC, Hart R, Golitsyn S, for the AVERROES Steering Committee and Investigators, et al. Apixaban in patients with atrial fibrillation. N Engl J Med. 2011;364:806–17.

15. APPRAISE Steering Committee and Investigators. Apixaban, an oral, direct, selective factor Xa inhibitor, in combination with antiplatelet therapy after acute coronary syndrome: results of the Apixaban for Prevention of Acute Ischemic and Safety Events (APPRAISE) trial. Circulation. 2009;119(22):2877–85.
16. Lopes RD, Alexander JH, Al-Khatib SM, Ansell J, Diaz R, Easton JD. Apixaban for reduction in stroke and other thromboembolic events in atrial fibrillation (ARISTOTLE) trial: design and rationale. Am Heart J. 2010;159(3):331–9.
17. Baetz BE, Spinler SA. Dabigatran etexilate: an oral direct thrombin inhibitor for thromboprophylaxis and treatment of thromboembolic diseases. Pharmacotherapy. 2008;28:1354–73.
18. Stangier J, Rathgen K, Staehle H, et al. The pharmacokinetics, pharmacodynamics and tolerability of dabigatran etexilate, a new oral direct thrombin inhibitor, in healthy male subjects. Br J Clin Pharmacol. 2007;64:292–303.
19. Di Nisio M, Middeldorp S, Buller HR. Direct thrombin inhibitors. N Engl J Med. 2005;353:1028–40.
20. Stangier J, Rathgen K, Stahle H, Reseski K, Körnicke T, Roth W. Coadministration of dabigatran etexilate and atorvastatin: assessment of potential impact on pharmacokinetics and pharmacodynamics. Am J Cardiovasc Drugs. 2009;9:59–68.
21. Stangier J, Stahle H, Rathgen K. No interaction of the oral direct thrombin inhibitor dabigatran etexilate and digoxin (abstract). J Thromb Haemost. 2007;5(52):P-W 672.
22. Pradaxa (dabigatran etexilate). Summary of product characteristics. Boehringer Ingelheim International GmbH. http://www.pradaxa.com/Include/media/pdf/Pradaxa_SPC_EMEA.pdf. (Accessed march 30th 2012)
23. Eriksson BI, Dahl OE, Rosencher N, Kurth AA, van Dijk CN, Frostick SP, RE-NOVATE Study Group, et al. Dabigatran etexilate versus enoxaparin for prevention of venous thromboembolism after total hip replacement: a randomized, double-blind, noninferioritytrial. Lancet. 2007;370:949–56.
24. Eriksson BI, Dahl OE, Rosencher N, Kurth AA, van Dijk CN, Frostick SP, et al. Oral dabigatran etexilate versus subcutaneous enoxaparin for the prevention of venous thromboembolism after total knee replacement: the RE-MODEL randomized trial. J Thromb Haemost. 2007;5:2178–85.
25. RE-MOBILIZE Writing Committee, Ginsberg JS, Davidson BL, Comp PC, Francis CW, Friedman RJ, Huo MH, et al. The oral thrombin inhibitor dabigatran etexilate vs the North American enoxaparin regimen for the prevention of venous thromboembolism after knee arthroplasty surgery. J Arthroplasty. 2009;2:1–9.
26. Schulman S, Kearon C, Kakkar AK, Mismetti P, Schellong S, Eriksson H. Dabigatran versus warfarin in the treatment of acute venous thromboembolism. N Engl J Med. 2009;361:2342–52.
27. Connolly SJ, Esekowitz MD, Yusuf S, et al. Dabigatran versus warfarin in patients with atrial fibrillation. N Engl J Med. 2009;361:1139–51.
28. Wann LS, Curtis AB, Ellenbogen KA, Estes 3rd NA, Ezekowitz MD, Jackman WM, et al. ACCF/AHA/HRS focused update on the management of patients with atrial fibrillation (update on dabigatran): a report of the American College of Cardiology Foundation/American Heart Association Task Force on practice guidelines. J Am Coll Cardiol. 2011;57(11):1330–7.
29. Oldgren J, Budaj A, Granger CB, Khder Y, Roberts J, Siegbahn A, for the RE-DEEM investigators, et al. Dabigatran vs. placebo in patients with acute coronary syndromes on dual antiplatelet therapy: a randomized, double-blind, phase II trial. Eur Heart J. 2011;32:2781. Epub ahead of print.
30. Kubitza D, Becka M, Voith B, Zuehlsdorf M, Wensing G. Safety, pharmacodynamics, and pharmacokinetics of single doses of BAY 59-7939 an oral, direct factor Xa inhibitor. Clin Pharmacol Ther. 2005;78:412–21.
31. Eriksson BI, Borris LC, Friedman RJ, Haas S, Himan MV, Kakkar AK, et al. Rivaroxaban versus enoxaparin for thromboprophylaxis after hip arthroplasty. N Engl J Med. 2008;358:2765–75.

32. Kakkar AK, Brenner B, Dahl OE, Eriksson BI, Mouret P, Muntz J, et al. Extended duration rivaroxaban versus short-term enoxaparin for the prevention of venous thromboembolism after total hip arthroplasty: a double-blind randomized controlled trial. Lancet. 2008;372:31–9.
33. Lassen MR, Ageno W, Borris LC, Lieberman JR, Rosencher N, Bandel TJ, RECORD 3 Investigators, et al. Rivaroxaban for thromboprophylaxis after total knee arthroplasty. N Engl J Med. 2008;358:2776–85.
34. Turpie A, Lassen MR, Davidson BL, Bauer KA, Gent M, Kwong LM, RECORD 4 Investigators, et al. Rivaroxaban versus enoxaparin for thromboprophylaxis after total knee arthroplasty (RECORD 4): a randomized trial. Lancet. 2009;373:1673–80.
35. Xarelto (rivaroxaban). Summary of product characteristics. Bayer Schering Pharma. http://www.xarelto.com. (Accessed march 30th 2012).
36. Kubitza D, Becka M, Zuehlsdorf M, Mueck W. Effect of food, an antacid, and the H2 antagonist ranitidine on the absorption of BAY 59–7939 (rivaroxaban), an oral, direct factor Xa inhibitor, in healthy subjects. J Clin Pharmacol. 2006;46(5):549–58.
37. The Einstein Investigators. Oral rivaroxaban for symptomatic venous thromboembolism. N Eng J Med. 2010;363:2499–510.
38. Patel MR, Mahaffey KW, Garg J, Pan G, Singer DE, Hacke W, the ROCKET AF Steering Committee, for the ROCKET AF Investigators, et al. Rivaroxaban versus warfarin in nonvalvular atrial fibrillation. N Engl J Med. 2011;365:883–91.
39. Vandermeulen EP, Van Aken H, Vermylen J. Anticoagulants and spinal–epidural anesthesia. Anesth Analg. 1994;79:1165–77.
40. Rosencher N, Bonnet MP, Sessler DI. Selected new antithrombotic agents and neuraxial anaesthesia for major orthopedic surgery: management strategies. Anaesthesia. 2007;62:1154–60.
41. Wulf H. Epidural anaesthesia and spinal haematoma. Can J Anaesth. 1996;43:1260–71.

Chapter 7
Effectiveness of Mechanical Devices in Orthopedic Surgery

David J. Warwick

Abstract Orthopedic surgeons are intuitively drawn to mechanical thromboprophylactic methods because of the perceived lack of bleeding complications, fear of which inhibits universal acceptance of effective chemical methods. Some mechanical methods such as graduated stockings, foot pumps, and calf compressors have a good evidence base with studies showing a consistent reduction in thrombosis. Drawbacks include cost, convenience, and compliance. The ideal role is in conjunction with, rather than in competition with, chemical methods.

Keywords Thromboembolism • Foot pumps • Graduated stockings • Intermittent pneumatic compression • Orthopedics

Introduction

Orthopedic surgeons rightly fear surgical bleeding – a complication that reflects on the perceived competence of their operation; many surgeons are understandably cynical about the true prevalence of symptomatic venous thrombosis (something which they rarely see). However, the very occasional embolic event can be catastrophic, and so thromboprophylaxis is strongly encouraged by many consensus groups such as the ACCP and ICS [1, 2] and government agencies such as NICE [3]. The risk to the surgeon of litigation is also a strong motivator to use prophylaxis. A recent meta-analysis through the UK NHS Health Technology Assessment process [4] reviewed 17 GCS trials, 22 IPC trials, and 3 foot pump trials. Of these, 14 trials were in hip and knee surgery. The review concluded a 72 % odds reduction for mechanical methods alone.

D.J. Warwick, M.D., FRCS, FRCS (Orth)
Department of Orthopaedic Surgery, University of Southampton,
Southampton SO16 6UY, UK
e-mail: davidwarwick@me.com

J.V. Llau (ed.), *Thromboembolism in Orthopedic Surgery*,
DOI 10.1007/978-1-4471-4336-9_7, © Springer-Verlag London 2013

Fig. 7.1 Virchow's triad

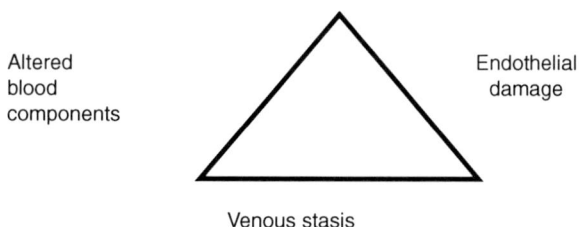

Against this background, mechanical methods are intuitively attractive to orthopedic surgeons. The evidence for these devices, the disadvantages, and their integration into an overall strategy for prophylaxis are discussed in this chapter.

Pathophysiology of Venous Stasis

Virchow's Triad

According to Virchow [5], there are three interrelating factors which predispose to venous thrombosis: altered blood components, venous stasis, and endothelial damage (Fig. 7.1).

While blood flows, the active coagulation enzymes are flushed away from the area of local endothelial damage to be cleared by reticuloendothelial cells; furthermore, while in transit, these enzymes are inhibited by plasma factors which are able to neutralize more coagulant enzymes than are present in the quantum of flowing blood [6].

Static blood is hypoxic. Hypoxic endothelium generates clotting factors and thromboplastins [7]. Venous stasis in valve pockets (the usual site of thrombus formation), for example, from femoral vein obstruction, leads to progressive hypoxia as the endothelium consumes oxygen. After 2 h of venous obstruction, the valve pocket pO_2 falls to zero. Pulsatile flow in the lumen returns the valve pocket pO_2 to normal [8].

Venous stasis provokes thrombosis by:

- Accumulation of clotting factors in the stagnant blood
- Hypoxia of venous blood
- Direct damage to endothelium by kinking during surgical manipulation
- Distension of valves, inhibiting venous return
- Distension of venous endothelium, exposing subendothelial collagen

Blood Flow

Blood flow is affected in various ways after orthopedic surgery:

- *Intraoperative occlusion*: During hip replacement, there is venous stasis which has been shown *indirectly* with venographic and cadaveric studies which show kinking of the femoral vein at the level of the greater trochanter [9–11]. Ultrasonic studies show reduced blood flow as the hip is dislocated and levers are placed around the acetabulum [12]. During knee replacement, there is likely to be reduced flow as the tibia is subluxated forward. Venous occlusion will cause distension of the veins in the leg, causing endothelial damage – a further component of Virchow's triad.

- *Postoperative immobility*: After a lower limb procedure, the patient will be unable to fully weight-bear for some period of time, denying them the usual physiological mechanism of emptying the plantar venous plexus through the deep venous system of the leg [13].
- *Plaster cast*: Many injuries and procedures require a plaster cast; this will reduce the function of the calf muscle pump and plantar venous plexus.
- *Physiological change*: Plethysmographic studies have shown that venous flow in the operated leg takes 6 days to recover after knee replacement and 6 weeks after hip replacement and hip fracture [14–16]. This matches the known risk period for thrombosis after each procedure although the mechanism is unclear.
- *Tourniquet*: The use of a tourniquet will stop venous return, causing an accumulation of clotting factors [17–19]. While there appears to be no effect on the DVT rate after knee replacement [20] (perhaps because the washout effect after deflation is fibrinolytic), it is concerning to note that embolic material can be seen entering the chest when the tourniquet is released [21].

Mode of Action of Mechanical Devices

Mechanic methods enhance venous return by various means [22]: emptying of the plantar plexus (foot impulse devices), reduction of venous capacity (graduated stockings), and emptying of the calf veins (sequential compression devices). Physiological studies of mechanical devices compare peak venous in the leg veins as a surrogate for efficacy [23].

Fibrinolysis

Mechanical methods also have a fibrinolytic effect [24–26]. There is probably a reduction in the antigen to tissue plasminogen activator (tPA) activity and an increase in plasminogen activator inhibitor (PAI-1) activity [27]. Intermittent compression increases euglobulin clot lysis time [28]. In addition, there is some evidence that prostaglandin and nitric oxide production is increased thus inhibiting platelet aggregation [29, 30]. There also appears to be reduced factor VIIa activity and increased tissue factor pathway inhibitor (TFPI) [31], supporting the theory that mechanical prophylaxis may actually inhibit thrombus formation.

Intriguingly, intermittent compression of the arm will reduce thrombosis in the legs after surgery, implying increased systemic fibrinolytic activity [32]. With mechanical devices, the rate of inflation may also be relevant, since rapid inflation and deflation affects fibrinolytic activity in healthy volunteers less than a slower cycle [28].

Simple Nonchemical Prophylaxis

Surgical Technique

Careless tissue handling potentiates thromboplastin release. Retractors in the acetabulum and torsion of the dislocated hip while reaming during hip replacement will cause venous occlusion and, similarly, retraction of the tibia during knee replacement. The time spent on these maneuvers must be minimized, and they should be performed as gently as possible.

Early Mobilization

In orthopedic patients, earliest mobilization will enhance functional recovery but will also probably reduce the risk of VTE for which there is plausible physiological premise, although rather weak scientific evidence. In a nonrandomized study of 109 uncemented hip replacements, those non-weight-bearing for 6 weeks had an ultrasound-derived DVT rate of 19 %, whereas those mobilized fully weight-bearing immediately had a 0 % rate. All patients had IPC and aspirin [33]. In another study of THR patients given LMWH prophylaxis, those mobilized on the seventh day had a 75 % venographic prevalence of DVT whereas those mobilized on the third day had a 25 % prevalence [34].

Neuraxial Anesthesia

Anesthetists keenly use these techniques (spinal or epidural anesthesia) as they reduce mortality and enhance perioperative analgesia [35]. Furthermore, neuraxial anesthesia also reduces the risk of VTE because of hemodynamic effects in the legs [36, 37]. A systematic review [4] of 929 patients in 11 randomized studies (3 TKR, 4 THR, 2 hip fracture surgery, 1 urology, 1 general surgery) showed a 53 % odds reduction for the rate of DVT (28 % regional anesthesia, 53 % general anesthesia). Specific hypotensive techniques may yet further reduce the risk after TKR and THR [38, 39]. Care must be taken when used alongside chemical prophylaxis, and appropriate guidelines must be followed [40].

Graduated Compression Stockings

These devices (GCS) apply a constant pressure to the limb which decreases as the stocking moves proximally promoting blood flow to the heart [41]. Nongraduated elastic stockings do not work so effectively [42]. In well-fitted stockings, the pressure decreases from about 18 mmHg at the ankle through 14 mmHg in the upper calf and 8 mmHg at the upper thigh [43]. The prevention of venous distension and accumulation of blood is possibly the main mode of action [44].

Stockings may be below knee or above knee. Above-knee stockings are perhaps more uncomfortable and awkward to fit with reviews suggesting an advantage for below-knee stockings [45].

The fitting of stockings is essential. In a study of the pressure interface in three leading brands of thigh-length stockings, 70 % of readings showed a reversed pressure gradient and only 30 % of readings were within 20 % of the ideal profile [46]. In another study of calf-length stockings, 54 % had a reversed pressure gradient and 98 % were not within 20 % of the ideal pressure. Furthermore, there was an increased DVT frequency with the reverse gradient (26 % against 6 %) [47]. It is clear that GCS must be of high quality, properly fitted, and frequently checked to replicate the optimistic performance in randomized trials.

In a meta-analysis of nine studies comprising 1,293 randomized patients (orthopedics and general surgery), the odds reduction for stockings was 66 % (21.1 % control, 8.6 % stockings) [4]. In a Cochrane analysis of seven randomized trials (four of which were orthopedic) comprising 1,027 patients, the odds reduction was 47 % (29 % control, 15 % stockings) [48].

Rhythmic Mechanical Devices

Mechanical devices fall into three groups:

- Passive movement of the ankle
- Intermittent pneumatic compression: active sequential massage of blood from distal to proximal along the leg.
- Foot pumps: active expression of blood from the plantar venous plexus

These devices produce a pulse of blood which moves proximally through the deep veins. This pulse can be readily measured with Doppler ultrasound over the posterior tibial, popliteal, and common femoral veins. The pulse is described by either its peak velocity or the increase in velocity over the resting velocity. Different devices produce different profiles with many variables to include the rate, pressure, duration, and sequence. A typical maximum velocity at the femoral vein with 40 mmHg applied would be 35–60 m/s (corresponding to an increase in flow 50–250 %) [28]. Higher pressures and more rapid compression will augment peak velocity further, but this may not be tolerable to the patient, but the optimal velocity for thromboprophylaxis is unknown.

Rhythmic mechanical devices have disadvantages to include discomfort, the noise of the compressor, the cost of the devices, and the inconvenience for patient and staff in applying and removing them in the postoperative period. A significant disadvantage is the lack of portability which precludes these devices from providing extended duration prophylaxis which is now mandatory after hip and knee replacement because of the long duration of VTE risk [49, 50].

There have been very few comparisons between one rhythmic device and another. The foot pump was compared with IPC in 124 major trauma patients, with an advantage for the IPC in reducing ultrasound-demonstrated DVT (25 %) (6.5 vs. 25 % $p=0.009$) [51]. With regard to comfort, in a crossover study, 24/35 preferred a foot pump and 7 preferred IPC. Seventy-three percent were satisfied with the foot pump and 55 % with IPC. This was reflected in 77 % compliance with the foot pump and 73 % for IPC [52].

Passive Ankle Movement

There are very few data on passive ankle devices, although physiological studies show that there is enhanced venous blood flow [53]. One study of 227 trauma patients compared LWMW alone and LMWH with a passive ankle device (Arthroflow). The ultrasonic DVT prevalence was 25 % in the LMWH group and only 3.6 % in the Arthroflow-LMWH group ($p=0.001$) [54].

Intermittent Pneumatic Compression

These devices have been available since the 1970s [55, 56]. They rhythmically express blood from the leg. The devices typically contain three or more bladders which are sequentially activated from distal to proximal by a pneumatic pump. They have been further refined in some designs to inflate the most distal chamber with a higher pressure then the next proximal and so on, mimicking the graduated compression stockings. The devices may be below knee or above knee. They may be secured with Velcro straps or with zips. While they are traditionally circumferential, there are newer "asymmetric" designs which reduce the size of the bladder by just positioning it posteriorly, with a non-distensible wrapper around the rest of the leg. This requires less compression and thus less noise and perhaps more comfort. In theory, this pattern may also more effectively empty the veins [57]. A randomized study of asymmetric rapid inflation versus circumferential IPC in 423 TKR patients found a 6.9 % ultrasound DVT prevalence in the asymmetric group and 15 % in the circumferential group. The addition of GCS has no additive effect [58].

A most recent design has use impulse compression (derived from foot pump devices) applied to the calf with encouraging augmentation of flow rate [59]. A pressure of 40 mmHg is needed to fully occlude the veins; most IPC devices compress at 40 mmHg for about 12 s each minute. There is a probable physiological advantage to more rapid inflation and higher pressures [60]. There are potential complications with IPC, to include ischemia [61] and peroneal nerve palsy [62], although modern designs should ensure that the popliteal fossa is not compressed.

Table 7.1 Knee replacement and intermittent pneumatic compression

Author	Date	Number	DVT	%
Hull [63]	1979	29	2	6
MacKenna [64]	1980	10	1	10
Lynch [65]	1988	307	31	11
Haas [66]	1990	36	8	22

Knee replacement and IPC: (Combined DVT rate 11% 95 % CI 8–14 %)

Table 7.2 Hip replacement and intermittent pneumatic compression (all studies show significant risk reduction)

Author	Control	No	DVT (%) control	DVT (%) IPC
Hartman [67]	Nil	104	19	9
Gallus [68]	Nil	90	53	35
Paiement [69]	Warfarin	158	17	13
Hull [70]	Nil	310	49	24
Bailey [71]	Warfarin	97	27	6
Kaempffe [72]	Warfarin	40	24	16
Francis [73]	Warfarin	201	31	27

The orthopedic literature shows that IPC significantly reduces DVT frequency after hip and knee replacement (Tables 7.1 and 7.2). Meta-analysis of IPC confirms efficacy across various procedures and specialities. Vanek [74] demonstrated that IPC reduced the DVT relative risk by 62 % compared with placebo, 47 % compared with stockings, and 48 % compared with unfractionated heparin. There were insufficient studies to compare with LMWH. In major orthopedic surgery, the relative risk reduction was 69 % compared with placebo and 29 % compared with warfarin. Roderick et al. [4] reviewed 19 studies with 2,255 randomized patients (orthopedics and general surgery) and objective diagnosis of DVT. There was a 26 % odds reduction for IPC (23.4 % control, 10.1 % IPC).

Foot Pumps

Foot pumps were developed to mimic the venous function of weight-bearing. When weight is placed on the sole, the plantar venous plexus (venae comitantes of the lateral plantar arteries) is emptied as the longitudinal plantar arch is stretched [13]. The device is designed therefore to apply rapid compression with a high pressure (130 mmHg) to the sole of the foot, with a duration of 3 s. The compression is applied with a bladder wrapped around the foot.

The mechanism requires preload of the plantar veins, and so the foot must be slightly dependent or at least straight, but not elevated [75]. The concomitant use of graduated stockings is counterproductive as they prevent the plantar plexus from refilling. A recent randomized study of 800 THR and TKR patients using foot pumps either with or without concomitant GCS found no difference in ultrasonic

Table 7.3 Foot pump and knee replacement

Author	Centre	Control	Control (n)	Control DVT (%) (total/ proximal)	Foot pump (n)	Control DVT (%) (total/ proximal)
Wilson [79]	London	Nil	32	69/19	28	50/0
Westrich [23]	New York	Nil[a]	83	59/14	81	27/0
Norgren [80]	Lund	LMWH	15	0/0	15	27/0
Blanchard [81]	Lausanne	LMWH	60	27/3	48	65/6
Warwick [82]	Bristol	Nil	89	54/0	99	57/4

[a]Control = aspirin; study group = aspirin + foot pump

Table 7.4 Foot pump and hip replacement

Author	Test	Control			Foot pump	
		Type	Number	DVT (%) Total/proximal	Number	DVT (%) Total/proximal
Bradley [83]	VG	Heparin[a]	44	27/25	30	7/7
Fordyce [84]	VG	Stockings	40	40/32	39	5/2
Santori [85]	US	Heparin	65	35/20	67	13/3
Warwick [86]	VG	LMWH	138	18/13	136	13/9
Pitto [87]	US	LMWH	100	6/2	100	3/3
Stannard [88]	US	Heparin + aspirin	25	20	25	0/0

[a]Control = heparin; study group = heparin + foot pump

DVT frequency but better compliance without GCS [76]. Patients seem to find the foot pump equally acceptable as LMWH [77]. New small portable devices may allow more prolonged use [78].

Foot pumps are fairly effective after knee replacement and quite possibly equivalent to LMWH after hip replacement (Tables 7.3 and 7.4).

Other Nonchemical Prophylaxis

Electrical Stimulation

Electrical stimulation has been described [89]. There are few data on efficacy, and there is discomfort for the conscious patient. Recently, a highly portable device with adjustable current and pulse frequency attached to the skin over the peroneal nerve has been devised. This shows impressive augmentation of flow in the leg, suggesting a role as a simple, comfortable, and effective ambulatory thromboprophylactic device. Direct electrical stimulation of the foot also looks promising [90].

IVC Filters

These are inserted percutaneously through the femoral, jugular, or basilic vein and lodged in the inferior vena cava. They are particularly popular in North America, with over 30,000 deployed each year [91]. The devices do not prevent thrombosis – indeed, the presence in the IVC may promote thrombosis; they merely catch an embolus and prevent it reaching the pulmonary circulation. There is a high complication rate to include death, and so their use should be restricted to very specific conditions where anticoagulation is contraindicated, yet the risk of embolism is high (e.g., a pelvic fracture patient who has already developed a leg DVT yet needs a major surgical reconstruction).

Filters can be permanent, temporary or retrievable. Temporary filters are anchored with a retrieval wire which risks infection. Retrievable filters have design features allowing dislodgement through a jugular approach.

Early complications include infection, air embolism vessel or organ penetration, and later complication (PE, IVC thrombosis, migration, and arteriovenous fistula).

The efficacy is unclear with no robust randomized evidence, and the devices used in a very-high-risk group. There is probably some benefit which must be to some extent offset by the complication rate [91].

Combination of Mechanical and Chemical Methods

Mechanical devices should not be regarded as an alternative to chemical prophylaxis, rather an option to be used instead in some patients or as well as in others. Combinations of chemical and mechanical methods can be used in various ways. This requires the art of medicine, balancing the risk of thrombosis and the risk of bleeding [92]. It also requires an appreciation that randomized trials and guidelines should only inform and not dictate clinical practice [93]. Mechanical methods avoid bleeding but cannot be used for more than a few days as compliance becomes an issue. Chemical methods if given too close to surgery will necessarily cause bleeding. However, they can be used for as long as the risk of thrombosis persists – often several weeks. The latest oral agents are particularly effective and convenient. Thromboprophylaxis should be individualized for every patient, based upon a careful risk assessment and using methods which are evidence based and generally supported by Consensus guidelines.

High Risk of Bleeding

For those with a particularly high bleeding risk, mechanical methods are used for longer and chemical methods delayed; the drug is started only when the bleeding risk has decayed in the individual patient. In a study of 224 patients with long bone fractures to receive either LMWH starting 24–48 h, post-injury or foot pumps started immediately with LMWH from day 5. An ultrasound was performed before discharge. Occlusive DVTs were more prevalent in the LMWH group (11.3 vs. 2.9 % $p = 0.025$) as were PE (2.1 vs. 0 %); wound complications were higher in the early LMWH group (22 vs. 19 %) [94].

In another study, Esklander et al. [95] randomized 44 hip fractures to receive pre-operative LMWH ($n = 21$) or IPC followed by delayed LMWH ($n = 23$). The investigators found a drier operative field for the sequential group; the DVT rate was equivalent (although the study was underpowered with a trend in favor of sequential).

High Risk of Thrombosis

For those with a particularly high risk of thrombosis, both mechanical and chemical methods should be used simultaneously for as long as possible. Once the mechanical device becomes cumbersome, the greater risk of thrombosis (provoked by the surgery) is diminishing, and so it can be discontinued.

There is ample evidence to show that a combination of heparin and mechanical methods enhances efficacy:

- Roderick et al. [4] systematically reviewed 12 randomized trials (6 orthopedics, 5 general surgery, 1 medical) in which heparin was used with or without mechanical prophylaxis (8 GCS, 3 IPC, 1 foot pump). There was a 53 % extra reduction in DVT, consistent across speciality and mechanical device.
- In a recent Cochrane systematic review, Kakkos [96] found 11 studies (6 randomized) (7,431 patients) comparing IPC alone with IPC and chemical prophylaxis. The combined method reduced symptomatic PE from 2.7 to 1.1 % (OR 0.39, 95 % CI 0.25–0.63) and symptomatic DVT from 4 to 1.6 % (OR 0.43, 95 % CI 0.24–0.76).
- Silbersack and colleagues [97] randomized 131 patients to have either LMWH and GCS or LMWH and IPC. DVT was diagnosed with ultrasound; the rate was 40 % for TKR and 14 % for THR in the LMWH-GCS group and % for both THR and TKR in the LMWH-IPC group. There was, however, a 25 % noncompliance rate with the IPC.
- Fuchs et al. [54] demonstrated in 227 randomized trauma patients that combining the Arthroflow passive motion device with LMWH reduced the ultrasound DVT frequency from 25 to 3.6 % ($p = 0.001$).
- The thromboprophylactic effect of both heparin and aspirin is significantly enhanced after THR by the addition of a foot pump (see Tables 7.3 and 7.4, Figs. 7.2 and 7.3) [83, 98].
- Eisele et al. [60] compared LMWH alone with LMWH and IPC in 1,803 randomized orthopedic patients. The ultrasonic DVT prevalence was 1.7 % in the LMWH group and 0.4 % in the combined group ($p = 0.007$).

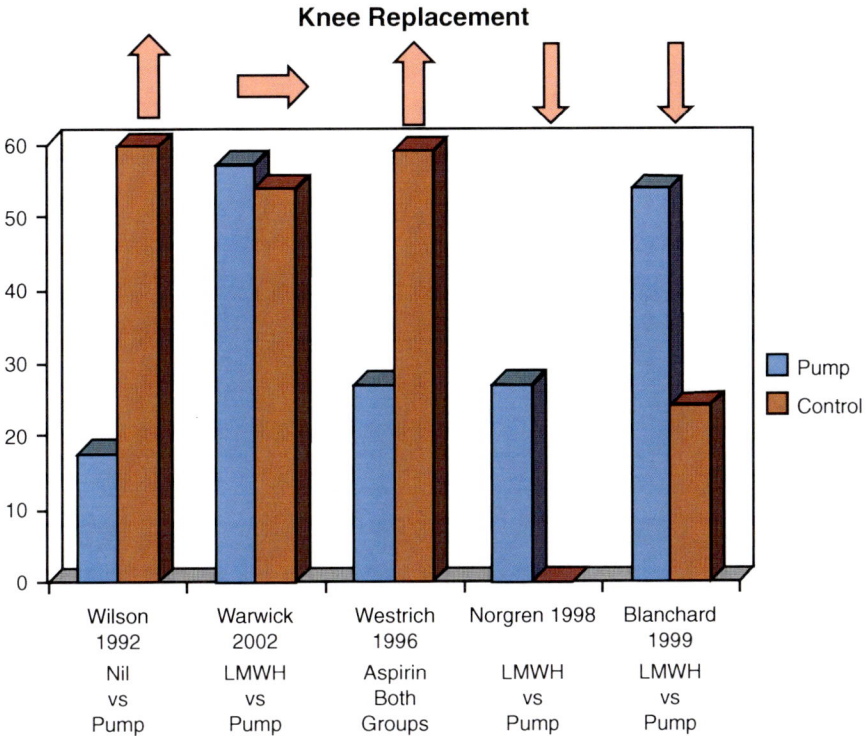

Fig. 7.2   Foot pump after knee replacement

- Edwards and colleagues [99] studied 277 THR and TKR patients randomized to either LMWH alone or LMWH with a new portable compression device. Patients were screened for DVT using duplex ultrasound at hospital discharge and followed clinically for 3 months. In TKA, the compression with LMWH group had 6.6 % DVT (ultrasound-diagnosed) compared with one pulmonary embolism and 19.5 % DVT rate in the LMWH group ($p = 0.018$). In THR, There was 1.5 % DVT compared with 3.4 %

Delay to Surgery

In some patients (especially hip fractures, pelvic fractures), there is an unpredictable delay to surgery because of the need to prepare the patient for surgery. Because surgery must not be performed too close to the administration of a chemical (due to the high bleeding risk), it may be safer to avoid chemical methods until after surgery. The mechanical method should be started as close to the moment of trauma as possible. If there is likely to be a prolonged delay, then a chemical can be started if there is no significant bleeding risk from the injury itself; the chemical will have to

Hip Replacement

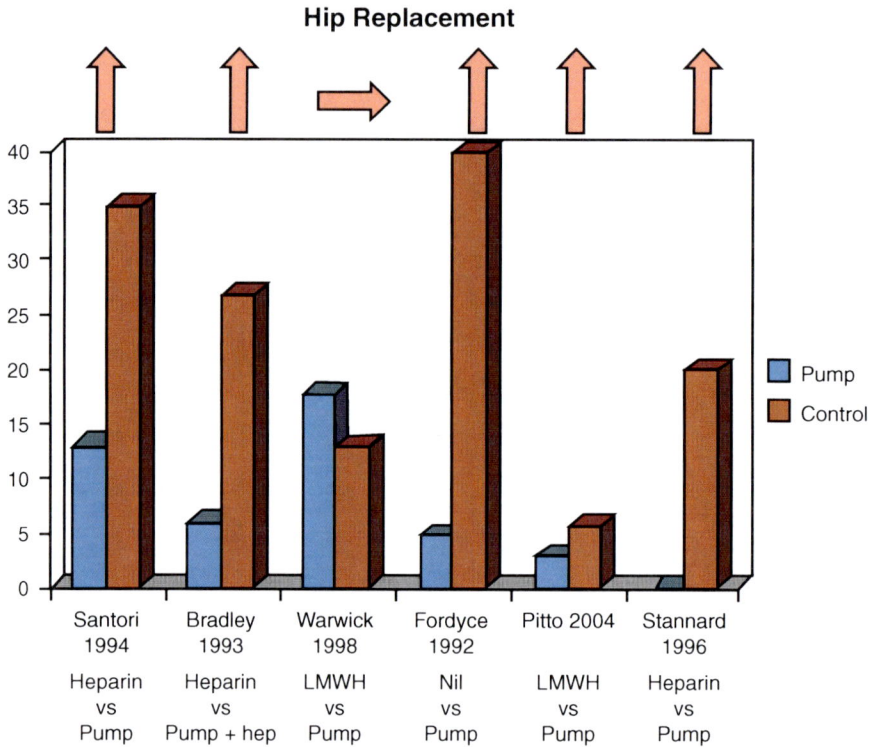

Fig. 7.3 Foot pump in hip replacement

be stopped and its bleeding effect allowed to decay until surgery is commenced. Again, mechanical methods provide cover during this interval but the surgery must be then delayed until the bleeding risk from the chemical itself has diminished.

Glossary

ACCP American College of Chest Physicians
DVT Deep vein thrombosis
GCS Graduated compression stockings
ICS International Consensus Statement
IPC Intermittent pneumatic compression
LMWH Low molecular weight heparin
NICE National Institute of Health and Clinical Excellence
PA Pulmonary embolism
THR Total hip replacement
TKR Total knee replacement
US Ultrasound
VTE Venous thromboembolism

References

1. Geerts WH, et al. Prevention of venous thromboembolism. The 8th ACCP conference on antithrombotic and thrombolytic therapy. Chest. 2008;133:381S–453.
2. Nicolaides AN, et al. Prevention and treatment of venous thromboembolism. International consensus statement (guidelines according to scientific evidence). Int Angiol. 2006;25(2):101–61.
3. NICE clinical guideline 92. Reducing the risk of venous thromboembolism (deep vein thrombosis and pulmonary embolism) in patients admitted to hospital. 2010. Available at: http://www.nice.org.uk/guidance. Accessed 10 Aug 2012.
4. Roderick P, Ferris G, Wilson K, Halls H, Jackson D, Collins R, Baigent C. Towards evidence based guidelines for the prevention of venous thromboembolism: systematic review of mechanical methods, oral anticoagulation, dextran and regional anaesthesia as thromboprophylaxis. Health Technol Assess. 2005;9(49):iii–iv, ix–x, 1–78.
5. Virchow RLK. Die verstopfung den lungenarterie und ihre flogen. Beitr Exper Path Physiol. 1846;2:227–380.
6. Wessler S, Yin ET, Gaston LW. A distinction between the role of precursor and activated forms of clotting factors in the genesis of venous thrombi. Thromb Diath Haemorrh. 1967;18:12–20.
7. Ogawa S, Gerlach H, Esposito C, Pasagian-Macaulay A, Brett J, Stern D. Hypoxia modulates the barrier and coagulant function of cultured bovine endothelium. J Clin Invest. 1990;85:1090–8.
8. Hamer JD, Lalone PC, Silver IA. The pO_2 in venous valve pockets: its possible bearing on thrombogenesis. Br J Surg. 1981;68:166–70.
9. Stamatakis JD, Kakkar VV, Sager S, Lawrence D, Nairn D, Bentley PG. Femoral vein thrombosis and total hip replacement. Br Med J. 1977;2:223–5.
10. Planès A, Vochelle N, Fagola M. Total hip replacement and deep vein thrombosis. J Bone Joint Surg Br. 1990;72-B:9–13.
11. Binns M, Pho R. Femoral vein occlusion during hip arthroplasty. Clin Orthop. 1990;255:168–72.
12. Warwick DJ, Martin A, Glew D, Bannister GC. Measurement of femoral vein blood flow during total hip replacement. Duplex ultrasound with and without the use of a foot-pump. J Bone Joint Surg Br. 1994;76-B:918–21.
13. Gardner AMN, Fox RH. The return of blood to the heart: venous pumps in health and disease. London: John Libby and Co; 2001.
14. McNally MA, Badahur R, Cooke EA, Mollan RA, et al. Venous haemodynamics in both legs after total knee replacement. J Bone Joint Surg Br. 1997;79:633–7.
15. McNally MA, Cooke EA, Mollan RA. Femoral vein blood flow during THR. J Bone Joint Surg Br. 1993;75:640–4.
16. Wilson D, Cooke EA, McNally MA, Yeates A, Mollan RA. Altered venous function and deep venous thrombosis following proximal femoral fracture. Injury. 2001;33:33–9.
17. Sharrock NE, Go G, Sculco TP, Ranawat CS, Maynard MJ, Harpel PC. Changes in circulatory indices of thrombosis and fibrinolysis during total knee arthroplasty performed under tourniquet. J Arthroplasty. 1995;10:523–8.
18. Sharrock NE, Go G, Williams-Russo P, Haas SB, Harpel PC. Comparison of extradural and general anaesthesia on the fibrinolytic response to total knee arthroplasty. Br J Anaesth. 1997;79:29–34.
19. Aglietti P, Baldini A, Vena LM, Abbate R, Fedi S, Falciani M. Effect of tourniquet use on activation of coagulation in total knee replacement. Clin Orthop. 2000;371:169–77.
20. Harvey EJ, Leclerc J, Books CE, Burke DL. Effect of tourniquet use on blood loss and incidence of deep vein thrombosis in total knee arthroplasty. J Arthroplasty. 1997;12:291–6.
21. Berman AT, Parmet JL, Harding SP, Israelite CL, Chandrasekaran K, Horrow JC, Singer R, Rosenberg H. Emboli observed with use of transesophageal echocardiography immediately after tourniquet release during total knee arthroplasty with cement. J Bone Joint Surg Am. 1998;80-A:389–96.

22. Von Schroeder HP, Coutts RD, Billings E, Mai MT, Aratow M. The changes in intramuscular pressure and femoral vein flow with continuous passive motion, pneumatic compressive stockings, and leg manipulations. Clin Orthop. 1991;266:218–26.
23. Westrich GH, Sculco TP. Prophylaxis against deep venous thrombosis after total knee arthroplasty. Pneumatic plantar compression and aspirin compared with aspirin alone. J Bone Joint Surg Am. 1996;78:826–34.
24. Ljungnér H, Bergqvist D, Nilsson IM. Effect of intermittent pneumatic and graduated static compression on factor VIII and the fibrinolytic system. Acta Chir Scand. 1981;147:657–61.
25. Jacobs DG, Piotrowski JJ, Hoppensteadt DA, Salvator AE, Fareed J. Hemodynamic and fibrinolytic consequences of intermittent pneumatic compression: preliminary results. J Trauma. 1996;40:710–6.
26. Comerota AJ, Chouhan V, Harada RN, Sun L, Hosking J, Veermansunemi R, Comerota Jr AJ, Schlappy D, Rao AK. The fibrinolytic effects of intermittent pneumatic compression: mechanism of enhanced fibrinolysis. Ann Surg. 1997;226:306–13.
27. Kessler CM, Hirsch DR, Jacobs H, MacDougall R, Goldhaber SZ. Intermittent pneumatic compression in chronic venous insufficiency favorably affects fibrinolytic potential and platelet activation. Blood Coagul Fibrinolysis. 1996;7:437–46.
28. Morris RJ, Woodcock JP. Evidence-based compression: prevention of stasis and deep vein thrombosis. Ann Surg. 2004;239:162–71.
29. Guyton DP, Khayat A, Husni EA, Schreiber H. Elevated levels of 6-keto-prostaglandin-F1α from a lower extremity during external pneumatic compression. Surg Gynecol Obstet. 1988;166:338–42.
30. Dai G, Tsukurov O, Chen M, Gertler JP, Kamm RD. Endothelial nitric oxide production during in vitro simulation of external limb compression. Am J Physiol Heart Circ Physiol. 2002;282:H2066–75.
31. Giddings JC, Morris RJ, Ralis HM, Jennings GM, Davies DA, Woodcock JP. Systemic haemostasis after intermittent pneumatic compression. Clues for the investigation of DVT prophylaxis and travellers thrombosis. Clin Lab Haematol. 2004;26:269–73.
32. Knight MT, Dawson R. Effect of intermittent compression of the arms on deep venous thrombosis in the legs. Lancet. 1976;2:1265–8.
33. Buehler KO, D'Lima DD, Petersilge WJ, Colwell CW, Walker RH. Late deep venous thrombosis and delayed weight bearing after total hip arthoplasty. Clin Orthop. 1999;361:123–30.
34. Lassen MR, Borris LC. Mobilisation after hip surgery and efficacy of thromboprophylaxis. Lancet. 1991;337:618.
35. Rodgers A, Walker N, Schug S, McKee A, Kehlet H, van Zundert A, et al. Reduction of postoperative mortality and morbidity with epidural or spinal anaesthesia: results from overview of randomised trials. BMJ. 2000;321:1493–7.
36. Modig J. Influence of regional anesthesia, local anesthetics and sympathicomimetics on the pathophysiology of deep vein thrombosis. Acta Chir Scand Suppl. 1988;550:119–27.
37. Knaggs AL, Delis KT, Mason P, Macleod K. Perioperative lower limb venous haemodynamics in patients under general anaesthesia. Br J Anaesth. 2005;94:292–5.
38. Sharrock NE, Haas SB, Hargett MJ, Urquhart B, Insall JN, Scuderi G. Effects of epidural anesthesia on the incidence of deep-vein thrombosis after total knee arthroplasty. J Bone Joint Surg Am. 1991;73-A:502–6.
39. Lieberman JR, Huo MH, Hanway J, Salvati EA, Sculco TP, Sharrock NE. The prevalence of deep venous thrombosis after total hip arthroplasty with hypotensive epidural anesthesia. J Bone Joint Surg Am. 1994;76-A:341–8.
40. Horlocker TT, Wedel DJ, Benzon H, Brown DL, Enneking FK, Heit JA, et al. Regional anesthesia in the anticoagulated patient: defining the risks (the second ASRA consensus conference on neuraxial anesthesia and anticoagulation). Reg Anesth Pain Med. 2003;28:172–97.
41. Lawrence D, Kakkar VV. Graduated, static, external compression of the lower limb: a physiological assessment. Br J Surg. 1980;67:119–21.
42. Rosengarten DS, Laird J, Jeyasingh K, Martin P. The failure of compression stockings (Tubigrip) to prevent deep venous thrombosis after operation. Br J Surg. 1970;57:296–9.

43. Jeffery PC, Nicolaides AN. Graduated compression stockings in the prevention of postoperative deep vein thrombosis. Br J Surg. 1990;77:380–3.
44. Coleridge-Smith PD, Hasty JH, Scurr JH. Deep vein thrombosis: effect of graduated compression stockings on distension of the deep veins of the calf. Br J Surg. 1991;78:724–6.
45. Ingram JE. A review of thigh-length vs knee-length antiembolism stockings. Br J Nurs. 2003;12:845–51.
46. Wildin CJ, Hui AC, Esler CN, Gregg PJ. In vivo pressure profiles of thigh-length graduated compression stockings. Br J Surg. 1998;85:1228–31.
47. Best AJ, Williams S, Crozier A, Bhatt R, Gregg PJ, Hui AC. Graded compression stockings in elective orthopaedic surgery. An assessment of the in vivo performance of commercially available stockings in patients having hip and knee arthroplasty. J Bone Joint Surg Br. 2000;82:116–8.
48. Amarigiri SV, Lees TA (2000) Elastic compression stockings for prevention of venous thrombosis. Cochrane Database Syst Rev. 2000;(3):CD001484.
49. Warwick D, Roschensher N. The "critical thrombosis period" in major orthopedic surgery: when to start and when to stop prophylaxis. Clin Appl Thromb Hemost. 2010;16(4): 394–405.
50. Warwick DJ, et al. Insufficient duration of venous thromboembolism prophylaxis after total hip or knee replacement when compared with the time course of thromboembolic events. J Bone Joint Surg Br. 2007;89B:799–807.
51. Elliot CG, Dudney TM, Egger M, Orme JF, Clemmer TP, Horn SD, Weaver L, Handrahan D, Thomas F, Merrill S, Kitterman N, Yeates S. Calf-thigh sequential pneumatic compression compared with plantar venous pneumatic compression to prevent deep-vein thrombosis after non-lower extremity trauma. J Trauma. 1999;47:25–31.
52. Robertson KA, Bertot AJ, Wolfe MW, Barrack RL. Patient compliance and satisfaction with mechanical devices for preventing deep venous thrombosis after joint replacement. J South Orthop Assoc. 2000;9(3):182–6.
53. Westrich GH, Specht LM, Sharrock NE, Windsor RE, Sculco TP, Haas SB, Trombley JF, Peterson M. Venous haemodynamics after total knee arthroplasty. Evaluation of active dorsal to plantar flexion and several mechanical devices. J Bone Joint Surg Br. 1998;80B:1057–106.
54. Fuchs S, Heyse T, Rudolfsky G, Gosheger G, Chylarecki C. Continuous passive motion in the prevention of deep vein thrombosis. J Bone Joint Surg Br. 2005;87B:1117–22.
55. Hills NH, Pflug JJ, Jeyasingh K, Boardman L, Calnan JS. Prevention of deep vein thrombosis by intermittent pneumatic compression of calf. BMJ. 1972;1:131–5.
56. Cotton LT. Intermittent compression of the legs during operation as a method of prevention of deep vein thrombosis. Proc R Soc Med. 1974;67:708.
57. Dai G, Gertler JP, Kamm RD. The effects of external compression on venous blood flow and tissue deformation in the lower leg. J Biomech Eng. 1999;121:557–64.
58. Keith SL, McLaughlin DJ, Anderson Jr FA, Cardullo PA. Do graduated compression stockings and pneumatic boots have an additive effect on the peak velocity of venous blood flow? Arch Surg. 1992;127:727–30.
59. Warwick DJ, Dewbury K. A novel approach to mechanical prophylaxis: calf impulse technology mimics natural ambulation more effectively than sequential calf compression. Int J Angiol. 2008;17:197–201.
60. Eisele R, Kinzle L, Koelsch T. Rapid-inflation intermittent compression for prevention of deep vein thrombosis. J Bone Joint Surg Am. 2007;89:1050–6.
61. Merrett ND, Hanel KC. Ischaemic complications of graduated compression stockings in the treatment of deep venous thrombosis. Postgrad Med J. 1993;69:232–4.
62. McGrory BJ, Burke DW. Peroneal nerve palsy following intermittent sequential pneumatic compression. Orthopedics. 2000;23:1103–5.
63. Hull R, Delmore TJ, Hirsh J, Gent M, Armstrong P, Lofthouse MMA, Blackstone I, Reed-Davis R, Detwiler RC. Effectiveness of intermittent pulsatile elastic stockings for the prevention of calf and thigh vein thrombosis in patients undergoing elective knee replacement. Thromb Res. 1979;16:37–45.

64. MacKenna R, Galante J, Bachmann F, Wallace DL, Kaushal SP, Meredith P. Prevention of venous thromboembolism after total knee replacement by high dose aspirin or intermittent calf and thigh compression. Br Med J. 1990;280:514–7.

65. Lynch AF, Bourne RB, Rorabeck CH, Rankin RN, Donald A. Deep-vein thrombosis and continuous passive motion after total knee arthroplasty. J Bone Joint Surg Am. 1988;70:11–4.

66. Haas SB, Insall JN, Scuderi GR, Windsor RE, Ghelman B. Pneumatic sequential compression boots compared with aspirin prophylaxis of deep vein thrombosis after total knee arthroplasty. J Bone Joint Surg. 1990;72A:27–31.

67. Hartman JT, Pugh JL, Smith RD, Robertson WW, Yost RP, Janssen HF. Cyclic sequential compression of the lower limb in prevention of deep vein thrombosis. J Bone Joint Surg. 1982;64A:1059–62.

68. Gallus A, Raman K, Darby T. Venous thrombosis after elective hip replacement. The influence of preventive intermittent calf compression and of surgical technique. Br J Surg. 1993;70:17–9.

69. Paiement G, Wessinger SJ, Waltman AC, Harris WH. Low-dose warfarin versus external pneumatic compression for prophylaxis against venous thromboembolism following total hip replacement. J Arthroplasty. 1987;2:23–6.

70. Hull RD, Rascob GE, Gent M, McLoughlin D, Julian D, Smithy FC, et al. Effectiveness of intermittent pneumatic compression for preventing deep vein thrombosis after total hip replacement. JAMA. 1990;263:2313–7.

71. Bailey JP, Kruger MP, Solano FX, Zajko AB, Rubash HE. Prospective randomised trial of sequential compression devices vs low-dose warfarin for deep venous thrombosis prophylaxis in hip arthroplasty. J Arthroplasty. 1991;6:S29–34.

72. Kaempffe FA, Lifeso RM, Meinking C. Intermittent pneumatic compression versus coumadin. Clin Orthop. 1991;269:89–97.

73. Francis CW, Pellegrini VD, Marder VJ, Totterman S, Harris CM, Gabriel R, Azodo MV, Leibert KM. Comparison of warfarin and external pneumatic compression in prevention of venous thrombosis after total hip replacement. JAMA. 1992;67:2911–5.

74. Vanek VW. Meta-analysis of effectiveness of intermittent pneumatic compression devices with a comparison of thigh-high to knee-high sleeves. Am Surg. 1998;64:1050–8.

75. Pitto RP, Hamer H, Kuhle JW, Radespiel-Troger M, Pietsch M. Haemodynamics of the lower extremity with pneumatic foot compression. Biomed Tech (Berl). 2001;46:124–8.

76. Pitto RP, Young S. Foot pumps without graduated compression stockings for prevention of deep-vein thrombosis in total joint replacement: efficacy, safety and patient compliance. A comparative, prospective clinical trial. Int Orthop. 2008;32(3):331–6.

77. Anand S, Asumu T. Patient acceptance of a foot pump device used for thromboprophylaxis. Acta Orthop Belg. 2007;73:386–9.

78. Froimson MI, Murray TG, Fazekas AF. Venous thromboembolic disease reduction with a portable pneumatic compression device. J Arthroplasty. 2009;24:310–6.

79. Wilson NV, Das SK, Kakkar VV, Maurice HD, Smibert JG, Thomas EM, Nixon JE. Thromboembolic prophylaxis in total knee replacement. J Bone Joint Surg. 1992;74B:50–2.

80. Norgren L, Toksvig-Larsen S, Magyar G, Lindstrand A, Albrechtsson U. Prevention of deep vein thrombosis in knee arthroplasty: preliminary results from a randomised controlled study of low molecular weight heparin vs foot pump compression. Int Angiol. 1998;17:93–6.

81. Blanchard J, Meuwly J-Y, Leyvraz P-F, Miron M-J, Bounameaux HP, Didier D, Schneider P-A. Prevention of deep vein thrombosis after total knee replacement. Randomised comparison between a low molecular weight heparin (nadroparin) and mechanical prophylaxis with a foot-pump system. J Bone Joint Surg. 1999;81B:654–9.

82. Warwick D, Harrison J, Whitehouse S, Mitchelmore A, Thornton M. A randomized comparison of a foot pump and low molecular weight heparin in the prevention of deep vein thrombosis after total knee replacement. J Bone Joint Surg. 2002;84B:344–50.

83. Bradley JG, Krugener GH, Jager HJ. The effectiveness of intermittent plantar venous compression in the prevention of deep venous thrombosis after total hip arthroplasty. J Arthroplasty. 1993;8:57–60.

84. Fordyce M, Ling RSM. A venous foot pump reduces thrombosis after hip replacement. J Bone Joint Surg. 1992;74B:45–9.
85. Santori ES, Vitullo A, Stopponi M, Santori N, Ghera S. Prophylaxis against deep venous thrombosis in total hip replacement. J Bone Joint Surg Br. 1994;76B:579–83.
86. Warwick DJ, Harrison J, Glew D, Mitchelmore A, Peters T, Donovan J. Comparison of the use of a foot pump with the use of low molecular weight heparin for the prevention of deep vein thrombosis after total hip replacement. J Bone Joint Surg. 1998;80A:1158–66.
87. Pitto RP, Hamer H, Heiss-Dunlop W, Kuehle J. Mechanical prophylaxis of deep-vein thrombosis after total hip replacement a randomised clinical trial. J Bone Joint Surg Br. 2004;86:639–42.
88. Stannard JP, Harris RM, Bucknell AL, Cossi A, Ward J, Arington ED. Prophylaxis of deep venous thrombosis after total hip arthroplasty by using intermittent compression of the plantar venous plexus. Am J Orthop. 1996;25:127–34.
89. Browse NL, Negus D. Prevention of postoperative leg vein thrombosis by electrical muscle stimulation. An evaluation with 125I-labelled fibrinogen. BMJ. 1970;3:615–8.
90. Czyrny JJ, Kaplan RE, Wilding GE, Purdy CH, Hirsh J. Electrical foot stimulation: a potential new method of deep venous thrombosis prophylaxis. Vascular. 2010;18:20–7.
91. Giannoudis PV, Pountos I, Pape HC, Patel JV. Safety and efficacy of vena cava filters in trauma patients. Injury Int J Care Injured. 2007;38:7–18.
92. Warwick DJ. New concepts in orthopaedic thromboprophylaxis. J Bone Joint Surg Br. 2004;86B:788–92.
93. Warwick DJ, Dahl OE, Fisher WD. Orthopaedic thromboprophylaxis: limitations of current guidelines. J Bone Joint Surg Br. 2008;90-B:127–32.
94. Stannard JP, Lopez RR, Volgas DA, Anderson ER, Busbee M, Karr DK, McGwin GR, Alonso JE. Prophylaxis against deep-vein thrombosis following trauma- a prospective randomized comparison of mechanical and pharmacologic prophylaxis. J Bone Joint Surg Am. 2006;88A:261–6.
95. Eskander MB, Limb D, Stone MH, Furlong AJ, Shardlow D, Stead D, Culleton G. Sequential mechanical and pharmacological thromboprophylaxis in the surgery of hip fractures. A pilot study. Int Orthop. 1997;21(4):259–61.
96. Kakkos SK, Caprini JA, Geroulakos G, Nicolaides AN, Stansby GP, Reddy DJ. Combined intermittent pneumatic compression and pharmacological prophylaxis for prevention of venous thromboembolism in high risk patients (a review). Cochrane Database Syst Rev. 2008;(4):CD005258.
97. Silbersack Y, Taute BM, Hein W, Podhaisky H. Prevention of deep vein thrombosis after total hip and knee replacement. J Bone Joint Surg Br. 2004;86B:809–12.
98. Westrich GH, Sculco TP. Prophylaxis against deep venous thrombosis after total knee arthroplasty. Pneumatic plantar compression and aspirin compared with aspirin alone. J Bone Joint Surg Am. 1996;78-A:826–34.
99. Edwards JZ, Pulido PA, Ezzet KA, Copp SN, Walker RH, Colwell Jr CW. Portable compression device and low-molecular-weight heparin compared with low-molecular-weight heparin for thromboprophylaxis after total joint arthroplasty. J Arthroplasty. 2008;23:1122–7.

Chapter 8
Anesthetic Implications of Thromboprophylaxis

Sibylle A. Kozek-Langenecker

Abstract Thromboprophylaxis increases the risk of bleeding – also the risk of spinal hematoma. Acute spinal compression can have dramatic consequences for the patients with lifelong neurological impairment. This chapter reviews the estimated incidences of spinal hematomas in different patient cohorts after lumbar and thoracic neuraxial anesthesia (1:480,000–1:3,600). In order to avoid spinal bleeding in high-risk patients receiving anticoagulant, antiplatelet agents, or both, recommendations have been prepared. In this chapter, recent guidelines of the European Society of Anaesthesiology (ESA), the Scandinavian Society of Anesthesiology and Intensive Care Medicine (SSAI) and the American Society of Regional Anesthesia (ASRA) will be discussed and compared. In all three guidelines, recommendations on time intervals before and after neuraxial intervention (blockade, catheter insertion, and removal) are derived from pharmacokinetic parameters of the antithrombotic agent (half-life, time to peak effect) and expert opinion. While recommended time intervals are comparable, gradings differ considerably.

Aggregated information on currently available antithrombotic agents including their pharmacology, indications and side effects, as well as perioperative anesthesiological considerations is reviewed. Among these practice points, postoperative surveillance is essential: Early radiological diagnosis and treatment of spinal hematoma (laminectomy) is required. To avoid ischemia, antithrombotic treatment must be resumed as soon as bleeding risks are under control.

Keywords Thromboprophylaxis • Spinal hematoma • Neuraxial anesthesia Guidelines • Patient safety • Anticoagulants • Platelet inhibitors

S.A. Kozek-Langenecker, M.D., Professor M.B.A.
Department of Anesthesia and Intensive Care, Evangelic Hospital Vienna,
Hans-Sachs-Gasse 10-12, Vienna 1180, Austria
e-mail: sibylle.kozek@aon.at

J.V. Llau (ed.), *Thromboembolism in Orthopedic Surgery*,
DOI 10.1007/978-1-4471-4336-9_8, © Springer-Verlag London 2013

Incidence of Neuraxial Hematoma

The risk of spinal hematomas is extremely low, but acute spinal compression can have dramatic consequences for the patients with lifelong neurological impairment (paraplegia) and for the anesthetist with self-reproach and lawsuit. Large surveys permitted the evaluation of frequencies of complications. Thirty-three spinal hematomas were detected in Sweden during a 10-year period among 1.260,000 spinal blocks and 450,000 epidural blocks [1]. Interestingly, 25 of 33 neurologic complications occurred in the second half of the observation period which may indicate increased vigilance and reporting or hazardous treatment of patients with increased bleeding risks. The frequency of spinal hematoma after epidural analgesia was calculated to be much lower in obstetrics (1:200,000–1:562,600) than in elderly female orthopedic patients under combined spinal epidural anesthesia (1:3,600) [1, 2]. Likewise, elderly women undergoing hip fracture surgery under spinal anesthesia had an increased risk of spinal hematoma (1:122,000) compared with all patients undergoing spinal anesthesia (1:480,000). Subsequent reports from various countries calculated even higher frequency rates of up to 1:2,700–1:19,505 [3–6]. Consistent in case series and surveys, the risk of hemorrhage is lowest in spinal anesthesia (1:160,000) and highest in catheter epidural anesthesia or combined spinal epidural anesthesia (1:18,000) [7]. One report indicated that hematoma may be more common after lumbar compared to thoracic epidural anesthesia [5], but according to the recent data of the German network for safety in regional anesthesia, the incidence was higher after non-obstetric thoracic epidural blocks (1: 8,550) compared to non-obstetric lumbar epidural blocks (1:13,000) [2]. Nearly half of all cases of bleeding occur during the removal of an epidural catheter; therefore, this procedure must be regarded as critical as catheter insertion [7].

Further risk factors for spinal hematoma include traumatic and difficult puncture conditions (e.g., due to pathologic lesion of the spine), vascular surgery, renal and hepatic impairment, as well as advanced age and female sex [8]. Age-related differences in the volume compliance of the vertebral canal have been observed: While an epidural blood patch was leaking through the intravertebral foramina in young individuals within few hours [9], the volume of local anesthetics produced neurological symptoms in an elderly [10]. Differences in the spread of the local anesthetic solutions between younger and elderly patients have been observed [11].

Although the numbers of incidence vary considerably between surveys and mathematical calculations, it can be concluded that spinal anesthesia has a lower estimated incidence for the elderly orthopedic population scheduled for lumbar neuraxial anesthesia (below 1:100,000) compared to epidural anesthesia or combined spinal epidural anesthesia (above 1:18,000).

Guideline Activity

The lack of guidelines, as well as preexisting or acquired coagulopathies (e.g., drug-induced), are also well-accepted risk factors for spinal hematoma [7]. In order to increase quality of care and patient safety, many national anesthesia societies

[12, 13] have published their recommendations on regional anesthesia in patients receiving anticoagulant, antiplatelet agents, or both. The Scandinavian Society of Anesthesiology and Intensive Care Medicine (SSAI) appointed a task force of experts to establish a Nordic consensus on recommendations for the best clinical practice in providing effective and safe central nervous blockades in patients with increased risk of bleeding [14]. In 2008, the European Society of Anaesthesiology (ESA) formed a guideline committee to oversee the production of evidence-based guidelines aimed at improving the practice of anesthesia and harmonization of clinical management throughout Europe. The ESA guideline 2010 is a systematically developed recommendation that may assist the clinician in decision making, specifically in timing regional anesthesia in the clinical setting of a pharmacologically increased risk of bleeding [15]. The American pendent is the guideline of the American Society of Regional Anesthesia and Pain Medicine (ASRA) with its third edition published in 2010 [16].

These three guideline activities were initiated in the desire to increase patient safety. Recommendations may be adopted, modified, or rejected according to the clinical requirements and constraints. The use of any of these recommendations does not guarantee prevention of neuraxial hematoma and perioperative thrombosis but improves risk stratification and awareness. Although intended as scientific guidelines, they might also assist in legal disputes.

All three guidelines share the same problem of low scientific evidence supporting the recommendations. Events are too rare to be studied in a randomized clinical trial. Recommendations derived from case reports or expert opinion is based on a low level of evidence (grade C). Observational and epidemiologic series have documented conditions for safe performance of central blocks in patients with anticoagulants which justify moderate levels of evidence (grade B). In the ASRA guideline, well-done observational series yielding very large risk reduction was categorized as grade B or even grade A evidence. However, with a complication as rare as spinal hematoma, randomized clinical trials justifying highest level of evidence (grade A) are not available. All three guideline recommendations are, therefore, mainly based on logic and pharmacology of the antihemostatic agents concerned. Guidelines are always subjected to revision as new evidence or experience becomes available.

The grade of recommendation indicates the strength and degree of consensus agreement among the task force of experts. This explains, for example, the high grade recommendation of 1A in the ASRA guideline to avoid neuraxial techniques in patients with coagulopathies and 1B for the daily review of the patient's medical record to determine the concurrent use of medications that affect other components of the clotting mechanisms.

Time Intervals for Drug Withdrawal

Routine coagulation tests are largely unaffected by antihemostatic drugs and are not helpful in the assessment of the bleeding risk. Therefore, time intervals for drug withdrawal have been implemented in clinical practice and guidelines rather than laboratory drug monitoring [12–16]. The smaller the amount prescribed and the longer the delay between administration and neuraxial intervention (blockade or removal of catheters), the lower the risk of hemorrhage. It is generally perceived that adhering strictly to the appropriate time intervals before and after the administration of antihemostatic drugs improves patient safety and reduces the risk of hematoma formation by timing neuraxial interventions at the lowest blood level (trough level) of the agent.

The recommended time limits from the last dose of a drug to neuraxial intervention are generally based on the plasma half-life of the drug. After two half-lives, only 25 % of pharmacodynamic efficacy is expected [17]. It takes about 6–8 h for a plug to solidify into a stable clot. The time limit from invasive intervention to the next dose is based on the calculation of 6–8 h – the time from intake of the drug to its peak effect or maximum plasma concentration [18].

Drug combinations or interactions as well as reduced (renal or hepatic) elimination alter pharmacokinetics significantly, limit the value of recommended withdrawal times, and increase the risk for bleeding. In these clinical situations, guidelines recommend to prolonging the time intervals. The SSAI guideline further recommends the monitoring of postoperative kidney function (serum creatinine) in elderly patients with indwelling neuraxial catheters during thromboprophylaxis requiring renal excretion [14]. Table 8.1 compares recommended time intervals of the three guidelines [14–16].

Interesting additional information aside from time intervals can be found in the recommendations: The SSAI guideline reviews the clinical benefits of central nervous blockade in surgical and obstetric patients [14]. Specifically, the effect on mobilization, patient comfort, morbidity, and mortality is outlined, as well as the differences between thoracic and lumbar epidural blocks. In the ASRA guideline [16], current recommendations on the prevention and treatment of venous thromboembolism are reviewed, and individual cases and case series are presented.

Points of Interest About Antithrombotic Drugs

Aside from recommending time intervals, the guidelines also aggregate information on currently available antihemostatic agents including their pharmacology, indications, and side effects.

Unfractionated Heparin

In the ASA closed claim analysis, spinal epidural hematoma occurred most frequently in vascular surgery patients, suggesting that this population is at an increased risk [18]. The ESA, ASRA, and SSAI guidelines state that the risk of hemorrhage after epidural anesthesia and subsequent intraoperative heparinization is not increased if heparinization is delayed for 1 h after puncture.

Table 8.1 Recommendations for time intervals before and after anticoagulant drug administration and neuraxial intervention (puncture or catheter removal)

Time interval	ESA		ASRA		SSAI	
	From drug intake to intervention	From intervention to next drug dose	From drug intake to intervention	From intervention to next drug dose	From drug intake to intervention	From intervention to next drug dose
Unfractionated heparin ≤5,000 U/day	4–6 h	1 h	2–4 h	1 h	4 h	1 h
Unfractionated heparin >5,000 U/day	i.v. 4–6 h s.c. 8–12 h	1–2 h Full heparinization: 6–12 h	Normal coagulation	1 h Bloody tap: 24 h	4 h	6-h (1–2 h common practice)
LMWH ≤40 mg/day enoxaparin	12 h	4 h	10–12 h Singe-daily dose and no additional drugs	2 h Before start of LMWH	10 h Emergencies: 0 h	6 h (2–4 h common practice)
LMWH >40 mg/day enoxaparin	24 h	4 h	24 h Twice-daily dose	Start 2 h after catheter removal	24 h	6 h (2–4 h common practice)
Fondaparinux ≤2.5 mg/day	36–42 h	6–12 h	Avoid catheters		36 h	6 h
Rivaroxaban ≤10 mg/day	22–26 h	4–6 h	Cautious approach		18 h	6 h
Apixaban ≤5 mg/day	26–30 h	4–6 h	Not mentioned		Insufficient data	6 h
Dabigatran ≤220 mg/day	Contraindicated according to the manufacturer		Cautious approach		Insufficient data	6 h
Argatroban	2 h	4 h	Insufficient data		Insufficient data	
Hirudins	8–10 h	2–4 h	Insufficient data		Insufficient data	
Vitamin K antagonists	INR ≤1.4	Restart after catheter removal	Normal INR	INR ≤1.5	INR ≤1.4(−2.2) 1–4 days	Restart after catheter removal

In the ESA guideline removal of epidural catheters should not be carried out until at least 4 h after the end of heparin administration with normalization of coagulation parameters (aPTT, ACT). Grading is different between the guidelines: Delay of indwelling neuraxial catheter removal for 2–4 h after the last heparin dose has grade 1A in the ASRA guideline, while the time interval of 4 h in the presence of normal aPTT and platelet counts has only a grade D in the SSAI guideline.

If a bloody puncture occurs in patients in whom intraoperative heparinization is planned, the ESA guideline recommends that low-dose anticoagulation (e.g., 5,000 IU) should be avoided for 1–2 h and full heparinization should be avoided for 6–12 h, with the operation being delayed to the next day if necessary. Alternatively, to avoid delays, epidural catheter placement can be carried out the evening before surgery. This is explicitly recommended by the ASRA guideline and in cardiac surgery using extracorporeal circulation [19]. In view of the limited benefits of neuraxial blockade in cardiac surgery, with no major effect on morbidity and mortality and considering the significant risks, it is disputable whether spinal and epidural techniques are justified at all or should be abandoned in this particular patient population [20].

Local dosing regimens are included in specific guidelines, for example, the ASRA guideline deals with thrice-daily dosing of subcutaneous unfractionated heparin.

Low-Molecular-Weight Heparins (LMWH)

A meta-analysis of studies on the timing of thromboprophylaxis showed that LMWH given 12 h preoperatively does not reduce the risk of thromboembolism compared with a postoperative regimen [21]. Since it is known that antithrombotic drugs increase the risk of spinal epidural hematomas after neuraxial blockade, a postoperative start may be advantageous.

All three guidelines give the following recommendation: To avoid bleeding complications, there should be a time interval of at least 10–12 h between subcutaneous administration of LMWH in prophylactic dosages and the placement or removal of a neuraxial catheter. In addition, the SSAI guideline recommends no time interval in emergency cases on LMWH 2,500 units or 20 mg twice daily if there is a strong indication for spinal anesthesia (because of a high benefit vs. risk balance, e.g., hip fracture, urgent cesarean section).

At a therapeutic dosage, neuraxial intervention should be delayed for at least 24 h after the last administration according to all three guidelines. Whether a 24-h interval is acceptable in relation to the thromboembolism risk needs to be considered on an individual basis. In cases at high risk of thromboembolism (e.g., mitral or double mechanical valve replacement), one should refrain from neuraxial blockade and continue the administration of LMWH.

An indwelling epidural catheter during single-daily dosing of LMWH is considered safe in Europe, but the American approach is much more conservative (owing to the large number of spinal hematoma after approval of LMWH in North America). Following neuraxial intervention, repeat administration of LMWH should be delayed for at least 2 h according to the ASRA guideline and for 4 h according to the ESA guideline. The SSAI guideline recommends 6 h but acknowledges that a 2–4 h time interval represents common clinical practice.

Anti-Xa levels are not predictive of the risk of bleeding. The ASRA guideline explicitly recommends against the routine use of laboratory drug monitoring.

Impaired bioavailability after subcutaneous administration of LMWH, for example, due to edema, hypoperfusion, hypothermia, and use of catecholamines, has been accused to reduce thromboprophylaxis in critically ill patients [22]. Modified resorption may be relevant to specific orthopedic patients and may change the time until trough levels are reached.

Fondaparinux

The EXPERT study with a total of 5,387 patients [23] used a time interval of 36 h before catheter removal and 12 h after catheter removal before the next dose of fondaparinux for thromboprophylaxis. These intervals have also been recommended by the ESA, while the SSAI recommends at least 6 h after catheter removal before the next intervention. The ASRA recommends against the use of indwelling neuraxial catheters.

In cases of therapeutic anticoagulation with fondaparinux (5–10 mg/day), neuraxial anesthesia should not be performed due to the substantial risk of accumulation according to ESA.

Anti-Xa levels standardized for fondaparinux may be used for drug monitoring (ESA).

Rivaroxaban

A time interval of 18–26 h between the last dose of rivaroxaban (10 mg) and puncture or catheter withdrawal is recommended [14, 16]. The ASRA task force only recommends a cautious approach. After catheter withdrawal, the next dose of rivaroxaban may be given after 4–6 h (ESA) and 6 h (SSAI). Prothrombin time or anti-Xa activity standardized for rivaroxaban may be used for drug monitoring.

Impaired bioavailability after peroral administration, for example, due to induction or inhibition of P-glycoprotein or the loss of the oral anticoagulant dose by postoperative nausea and vomiting (PONV), may reduce the quality of thromboprophylaxis. Accordingly, perioperative anesthetic management needs to avoid PONV especially in this group of patients.

Apixaban

Although not in clinical use until its publication, the ESA guideline already extrapolated time intervals from pharmacologic data. Apixaban is not mentioned in the

ASRA guideline, and the SSAI task force acknowledges that there are not enough data available but suggest a time interval of 6 h after blockade or catheter manipulation and next drug administration.

Argatroban

Patients with acute heparin-induced thrombocytopenia frequently suffer from multiple organ failure including coagulation disturbances, making neuraxial blockade not advisable. A time interval of 4 h between the last dose of argatroban and puncture or catheter withdrawal and a time interval of 2 h until the next argatroban dose are recommended by the ESA. The ASRA recommends against the performance of neuraxial techniques in patients receiving thrombin inhibitors, and SSAI acknowledges that there are not enough data available.

The aPTT and ecarin clotting time (ECT), which is more specific, can be used with therapeutic doses of thrombin inhibitors (ESA).

Hirudins (lepirudin, desirudin) and heparinoids are also mentioned in the guidelines, but their clinical use is dramatically reduced due to the availability of safer alternative anticoagulation with reversible direct thrombin inhibitors.

Dabigatran

The manufacturer advises against the use of dabigatran in the presence of neuraxial blockade. This warning has medicolegal consequences, if a spinal epidural hematoma occurs. Although management is based on labeling precautions, theoretically, a time interval of 34 h between the last dose of dabigatran and puncture or catheter withdrawal can be extrapolated from pharmacokinetic data (ESA). ASRA only recommends a cautious approach. SSAI task force group concludes that there are insufficient data for preparing a recommendation but suggest a time interval of 6 h after blockade or catheter manipulation and next drug administration although the manufacturer states that the first dose should wait a minimum of 2 h after catheter removal.

Vitamin K Antagonists (Phenprocoumon, Warfarin)

In most of the countries, vitamin K antagonists are not used for thromboprophylaxis. Therapeutic anticoagulation with vitamin K antagonists represents an absolute contraindication to neuraxial blockade, and vitamin K antagonists should only be administered after the catheter has been removed. ESA and SSAI recommend to using a drug monitoring and perform a central nervous block at the international normalized ratio (INR) is ≤1.4. Neurologic assessment should be continued for at least 24 h after catheter removal (ASRA, grade 2C).

Platelet Inhibitors

Platelet inhibitors are not used for thromboprophylaxis. Nevertheless, due to the clinical relevance in elderly patients with cardiovascular comorbidities scheduled for major orthopedic surgery and regional blocks, implications of these drugs on anesthetic and analgesic strategies are also briefly reviewed in this chapter. For more details for the "full" management of platelet inhibitors, refer to the Chap. 12.

Nonsteroidal Anti-inflammatory Drugs (NSAIDs)

On the basis of the available data, it can be assumed that NSAIDs by themselves do not lead to an increased risk of spinal epidural hematomas [24–26] and thus do not represent a contraindication in the ESA guideline. Similarly, the ASRA guideline recommends a liberal approach: There are no concerns as to the timing of single shot or catheter techniques in patients on NSAIDs (grade 1A). On the contrary, SSAI recommends a conservative approach in patients on systemic therapy with NSAIDs with time intervals before central blockade or catheter removal of 12 h (e.g., diclofenac, ibuprofen) to 2 days (e.g., piroxicam, tenoxicam) depending on the half-life of the drug (grade D). NSAIDs can be started or restarted about 1 h after intervention (grade D). Only after intra-articular administration and in emergencies with a strong indication for a central nervous blockade, no time interval is required according to the SSAI guideline. The authors of the SSAI guideline recommend that a nonselective NSAID should be replaced by another analgesic non-opioid drug (such as paracetamol or a selective COX-2 inhibitor) in the immediate perioperative period in patients planned for central blockade. The explanation for the discrepancies between the guidelines may be the difference in weighting several case reports indicating an association between NSAIDs and spinal hematoma [27–29].

Acetylsalicylic Acid (ASA), Thienopyridines, and Other Platelet Inhibitors

On the basis of the available data, it can be assumed that ASA by itself does not lead to an increased risk of spinal epidural hematomas [24–26] and thus does not represent a contraindication. A higher rate of complications has been observed in both surgical and medical patients when heparins were administered simultaneously [8]. Similar to the work-up of NSAIDs, the SSAI recommends to a restrictive strategy: In patients on ASA for secondary prevention after a coronary event, treatment should be continued up to the day before surgery and a planned central block. ASA treatment should be restarted as soon as possible after surgery (grade III/C). In patients on ASA for primary prevention of arterial thrombotic events, the authors of the SSAI guideline recommend that treatment should be interrupted for 3 days. In patients on higher doses of ASA (such as for analgesic or anti-inflammatory effects), 7 days should be allowed to elapse between the last ASA dose and a central block-ade. In emergency cases, patients on ASA may receive a central blockade provided there is a strong indication for it. In these cases, a single-shot spinal anesthesia is the preferred technique. The Nordic guideline reminds to considering reversal of the antihemostatic effects of ASA with desmopressin (and/or tranexamic acid).

Recommended time intervals for clopidogrel are consistently 7 days before neuraxial intervention. For ticlopidine, 10 days (ESA) to 14 days (ASRA) have been recommended. Restart of conventional thienopyridines is recommended after cath-eter removal.

Only the ESA guideline suggests time intervals for new platelet inhibitors: Neuraxial regional anesthesia should only be carried out if a time interval of 7–10 days between the last intake of prasugrel and the neuraxial intervention is possible. Restart of prasugrel appears possible 6 h after blockade or catheter removal. For ticagrelor, a pause of 5 days has been suggested, for cilostazol of 42 h (ESA).

Glycoprotein IIb/IIIa inhibitors and antiaggregatory prostaglandins are also mentioned in the guidelines. The clinical use of such agents is mainly limited to acute coronary syndromes. If a catheter has to be removed after unplanned glyco-protein IIb/IIIa administration, the ESA recommends waiting at least 48 h after abciximab and 8–10 h after tirofiban or eptifibatide.

Peripheral Nerve Blocks

Peripheral nerve blocks are more and more performed for orthopedic surgery. The recommendations for the management of anticoagulant drugs in this scenario are similar to those seen previously, but they have some particularities which is interest-ing to review.

The ASRA guideline summarizes cases and case series on bleeding complica-tions after peripheral nerve blocks and recommends a conservative approach for the management of patients on vitamin K antagonists and peripheral nerve blocks: Time intervals defined for neuraxial techniques should be applied (grade 1C). The ESA guideline, however, considers that peripheral nerve blocks cause less serious com-plications and are devoid of the risk of spinal hematoma and permanent neurologic damage; blood loss and transfusion requirements may be more serious than neural ischemia. Peripheral nerve blocks have been divided into two groups according to their bleeding risk and the access to a potential bleeding site [13]. Performance of superficial peripheral nerve blocks such as axillary plexus block, femoral nerve block, or distal sciatic nerve block is not contraindicated in the presence of antihemostatic agents if there is a normal bleeding history. However, for deep peripheral nerve blocks (close to vessels that cannot be compressed such as infraclavicular nerve block and lumbar sympathetic blockade), time intervals established for neuraxial blockade may be followed. The use of ultrasound-guided peripheral regional anesthesia helps avoiding vessel trauma and may shorten the recommended withdrawal intervals of anticoagulant and antiplatelet agents.

Anesthetic Implications Beyond Time Intervals

Preoperative Period

Anesthetists are increasingly confronted with patients who are being treated with highly effective and new anticoagulant medications or inhibitors of platelet function. Although not explicitly mentioned in the three management guidelines reviewed in this chapter [14–16], patient assessment including the drug history is an important instrument for detecting the involvement of antihemostatic drugs. Preoperative patient assessment (using standardized questionnaires), risk stratification, and planning of the anesthetic care are key elements in the perioperative process management which should be performed well in advance of elective surgical procedures in order to have time for further logistic, diagnostic, and therapeutic consequences. An example for a logistic consequence is the choice of anesthetic technique and individual timing of surgery and nerve blockade. A diagnostic consequence is performance of appropriate laboratory drug monitoring. An example of a therapeutic consequence is optimization of coagulation by procoagulant interventions.

The final decision to perform regional anesthesia in patients requiring drugs that affect hemostasis has to be taken after stratification of the individual risk and benefit. If it is judged that the administration of the anticoagulant must not be interrupted, an alternative anesthetic technique should be used (e.g., general anesthesia).

Preoperatively, patients need to be informed about the benefits and risks of the planned anesthetic procedure and potential anesthetic alternatives and finally give their written informed consent. For medicolegal reasons, patients have to be informed about frequent risks and – depending on the patient's will, reasonability, and national law – about the most severe adverse outcomes even if very rare.

Preoperative patient information should also include the significance of leg weakness and loss of sensation in the perineum as warning signs of spinal hematoma.

New anticoagulants may require new laboratory tests for sensitive monitoring. Instead of relying on the black box of nonindividualized time intervals, drug monitoring may help to individualizing perioperative patient management in the future.

Intraoperative Period

In order to minimize bleeding complications of regional anesthetic techniques, care should be taken to avoid a traumatic puncture. Patients with increased bleeding risks but an indication for neuraxial blockade should be treated by well-experienced anesthetists.

Postoperative Period

Spinal hematoma can occur late after surgery [30]. After performance of the block, the patient should be monitored at least until the effect of the regional anesthesia is clearly declining, that is, when there is a reduction in the extent of sensory block by two segments or a return of motor function. Particular attention should be given to persistent or progressing sensory or motor block and bowel/bladder dysfunction. Assessment is recommended every 4 h during ongoing epidural analgesia and for 24 h after removal of the catheter (SSAI). Radicular back pain and pressure sensitivity in the puncture area were not presenting symptoms of spinal hematoma [7]. The presence of postoperative numbness or weakness may misleadingly be attributed to local anesthetic effects rather than spinal hematoma which may delay diagnosis and timely correction. Accordingly, the lowest effective concentration of local anesthetic is recommended for postoperative (continuous) catheter techniques, and routine involvement of an acute pain service is advisable.

When there is a clinical suspicion of neuraxial hematoma, appropriate diagnostic (MRI, alternatively CT) or treatment measures (decompressive laminectomy) must be started before 6 to 12 h [7].

It is important to remember that antihemostatic agents are prescribed because of a risk of thrombotic manifestations. After drug withdrawal, surveillance for postoperative thrombosis or ischemia is essential during the postoperative recovery period, especially in patients receiving antiplatelet therapy. An early resumption of treatment postoperatively is essential.

References

1. Moen V, Dahlgren N, Irestedt L. Severe neurological complications after central neuraxial blockades in Sweden 1990-1999. Anesthesiology. 2004;101:950–9.
2. Vogt T, Wolf A, Van Aken H, et al. Incidence of spinal haematoma after epidural puncture: analysis from the German network for safety in regional anesthesia. Eur J Anaesthesiol. 2012;29:170–6.
3. Cameron CM, Scott DA, McDonald WM, Davies MJ. A review of neuraxial epidural morbidity: experience of more than 8,000 cases at a single teaching hospital. Anesthesiology. 2007;106:997–1002.

4. Christie IW, McCabe S. Major complications of epidural analgesia after surgery: results of a six-year survey. Anaesthesia. 2007;62:335–41.
5. Pöpping DM, Zahn PK, Van Aken HK, et al. Effectiveness and safety of postoperative pain management: a survey of 18 925 consecutive patients between 1998 and 2006 (2nd revision): a database analysis of prospectively raised data. Br J Anaesth. 2008;101:832–40.
6. Cook TM, Counsell D, Wildsmith JA. Major complications of central neuraxial block: report on the Third National Audit Project of the Royal College of Anaesthetists. Br J Anaesth. 2009;102:179–90.
7. Vandermeulen EP, Van Aken H, Vermylen J. Anticoagulants and spinal-epidural anesthesia. Anesth Analg. 1994;79:1165–77.
8. Stafford-Smith M. Impaired haemostasis and regional anaesthesia. Can J Anaesth. 1996;43: R129–35.
9. Beards SC, Jackson A, Griffiths AG, Horsman EL. Magnetic resonance imaging of extradural blood patches: appearance from 30 min to 18 h. Br J Anaesth. 1993;71:182–8.
10. Jacob AK, Borowiek JC, Long TR, et al. Transient profound neurologic deficit associated with thoracic epidural analgesia in an elderly patient. Anesthesiology. 2004;101:1480–1.
11. Usubiaga JE, Wikinski JA, Usubiaga LE. Epidural pressure and its relation to spread of anesthetic solutions in epidural space. Anesth Analg. 1967;46:440–6.
12. Llau VJ, De Andres J, Gomar C, et al. Anticlotting drugs and regional anaesthetic and analgesic techniques: comparative update of the safety recommendations. Eur J Anaesthesiol. 2007;24:387–98.
13. Kozek-Langenecker SA, Fries D, Gütl M, et al. Empfehlung der lokoregionalanästhesien unter gerinnungshemmender Medikation. Empfehlung der Arbeitsgruppe Perioperative Gerinnung (AGPG) der Österreichischen Gesellschaft für Anästhesiologie und Intensivmedizin (ÖGARI). Anaesthesist. 2005;54:476–84.
14. Breivik H, Bang U, Jalonen J, et al. Nordic guidelines for neuraxial blocks in disturbed haemostasis from the Scandinavian Society of Anaesthesiology and Intensive Care Medicine. Acta Anaesthesiol Scand. 2010;54:16–41.
15. Gogarten W, Vandermeulen E, Van Aken H, et al. Regional anaesthesia and antithrombotic agents: recommendations of the European Society of Anaesthesiology. Eur J Anaesthesiol. 2010;27:999–1015.
16. Horlocker TT, Wedel DJ, Rowlingson JC, et al. Regional anesthesia in the patient receiving antithrombotic or thrombolytic therapy. American Society of Regional Anesthesia and Pain Medicine evidence-based guidelines (third edition). Reg Anesth Pain Med. 2010;35: 64–101.
17. Rosencher N, Bonnet MP, Sessler D. Selected new antithrombotic agents and neuraxial anaesthesia for major orthopaedic surgery. Anaesthesia. 2007;62:1154–60.
18. Lee LA, Posner KL, Domino KB, Caplan RA, Cheney FW. Injuries associated with regional anesthesia in the 1980s and 1990s. A closed claims analysis. Anesthesiology. 2004;101: 143–52.
19. Chaney MA. Intrathecal and epidural anesthesia and analgesia for cardiac surgery. Anesth Analg. 1997;84:1211–21.
20. Chaney MA. Cardiac surgery and intrathecal/epidural techniques: at the crossroads? Can J Anaesth. 2005;52:783–8.
21. Strebel N, Prins M, Agnelli G, Büller HR. Preoperative or postoperative start of prophylaxis for venous thromboembolism with low-molecular-weight heparin in elective hip surgery. Arch Intern Med. 2002;162:1451–6.
22. Fries D. Thrombosis prophylaxis in critically ill patients. Wien Med Wochenschr. 2011;161: 68–72.
23. Singelyn FJ, Verheyen CCPM, Piovella F, et al. The safety and efficacy of extended thromboprophylaxis with fondaparinux after major orthopedic surgery of the lower limb with or without a neuraxial or deep peripheral nerve catheter: the EXPERT study. Anesth Analg. 2007;105:1540–7.

24. CLASP Collaborative Group (Collaborative Low-dose Aspirin Study in Pregnancy). A randomized trial of low dose aspirin for the prevention and treatment of pre-eclampsia among 9364 pregnant women. Lancet. 1994;343:619–29.
25. Horlocker TT, Wedel DJ, Schroeder DR, et al. Preoperative antiplatelet therapy does not increase the risk of spinal hematoma associated with regional anesthesia. Anesth Analg. 1995;80:303–9.
26. Horlocker TT, Bajwa ZH, Ashraf Z, et al. Risk assessment of hemorrhagic complications associated with nonsteroidal antiinflammatory medications in ambulatory pain clinic patients undergoing epidural steroid injection. Anesth Analg. 2002;95:1691–7.
27. Gerancher JC, Waterer R, Middleton J. Transient paraparesis after postdural puncture spinal hematoma in a patient receiving ketorolac. Anesthesiology. 1997;86:490–4.
28. Gilbert A, Owens BD, Mulroy MF. Epidural hematoma after outpatient epidural anesthesia. Anesth Analg. 2002;94:77–8.
29. Williams KN, Jackowski A, Evans PJD. Epidural haematoma requiring decompression following repeated cervical epidural steroid injection for chronic pain. Pain. 1990;42:197–9.
30. Moussallem C, El-Yahchouchi C, Charbel A, Nohra G. Late spinal subdural haematoma after spinal anaesthesia for total hip replacement. J Bone Joint Surg Br. 2009;91:B1531–2.

Chapter 9
Thromboprophylaxis in High-Risk Orthopedic Surgery: Total Hip and Knee Arthroplasty and Hip Fracture

Juan V. Llau and Raquel Ferrandis

Abstract Major orthopedic surgeries, mainly total hip or knee arthroplasty and hip fracture surgery, are procedures related with a high risk to develop venous thromboembolism. In patients scheduled for any of this types of surgery, it is mandatory to give pharmacological thromboprophylaxis, and it is probably recommended to add mechanical devices to increase its efficacy.

Although all the clinicians agree with previous statements, the controversies about the best drug, the optimal moment to begin the thromboprophylaxis, its duration, the real efficacy of the combination of both pharmacological and mechanical methods etc., are not solved. In this chapter, we review the most recent recommendations in this field, highlighting the most important recommendations in one of the most controversial scenario: the hip fracture surgery.

Keywords Total hip arthroplasty • Total knee arthroplasty • Hip fracture surgery Thrombotic risk • Thromboprophylaxis

J.V. Llau, M.D., Ph.D. (✉)
Department of Anesthesiology and Critical Care, Hospital Clínic Universitari de València,
Avda Blasco Ibáñez 17, 46006 Valencia, Spain

Human Physiology and Anaesthesiology, School of Medicine,
Catholic University "San Vicente Martir",
Valencia, Spain
e-mail: juanvllau@gmail.com

R. Ferrandis, M.D., Ph.D.
Department of Anesthesiology and Critical Care, Hospital Clinic Universitari de València,
Avda Blasco Ibáñez 17, 46006 Valencia, Spain

Human Physiology Department,
School Of Medicine, Valencia University, Valencia, Spain
e-mail: raquelferrandis@gmail.com

J.V. Llau (ed.), *Thromboembolism in Orthopedic Surgery*,
DOI 10.1007/978-1-4471-4336-9_9, © Springer-Verlag London 2013

Introduction

Patients undergoing major orthopedic surgery procedures as total hip and knee arthroplasty (THA and TKA) and hip fracture surgery (HFS) have a particular high risk to develop venous thromboembolism (VTE) in the perioperative period, and routine thromboprophylaxis has been included as standard care for them for many years [1].

The rates of VTE detected by venography, if no pharmacological prophylaxis is administered, range between 40 and 60 %, and this unacceptable incidence has been reduced until a symptomatic VTE rate ranging between 1.3 and 10 % within 3 months after surgery in patients receiving appropriate thromboprophylaxis [1]. This affirmation is supported by several meta-analyses which indicate that the administration of pharmacological thromboprophylaxis reduces the VTE rate with no relevant increase of bleeding risk [2].

One important challenge of these patients is the high rate of VTE after hospital discharge (during at least 2 months after surgery). This situation places us to recommend the extension of thromboprophylaxis at home, although the exact time for this extension is a major cause of debate.

So, at present, mechanical and/or pharmacological thromboprophylaxis is offered and performed in the vast majority of patients scheduled for any major orthopedic surgery procedure and, of course, in patients operated of THA, TKA, or HFS.

Methods for Thromboprophylaxis

The type of prophylaxis we can offer to these patients can be divided in:

- *General measures*, including mobilization and leg exercises. Adequate hydration should be ensured in immobilized patients.
- *Mechanical methods* increase mean flow velocity in leg veins and reduce venous stasis. They include graduated compression stockings (GCS), intermittent pneumatic compression (IPC) devices, and pneumatic foot pumps (PFP). Although they are included in most guidelines, GCS efficacy has been recently challenged in medical patients.
- *Pharmacological methods* are necessary when the thrombotic risk is moderate to high. They include low-molecular-weight heparins (LMWH) which are the most extended drugs used for thromboprophylaxis. Other drugs are fondaparinux, unfractionated heparin (UFH), anti-vitamin k (VKAs) (warfarin/acenocumarol) and new oral anticoagulants with direct action against factor Xa (apixaban and rivaroxaban) or against factor IIa (dabigatran). Among them, new oral anticoagulants are as effective, even more in some cases, but they could have the challenge to increase the bleeding risk in some fragile patients. The choice of the drug depends on several factors as the level of recommendation for each drug in each

Table 9.1 Suggested daily doses for thromboprophylaxis in patients scheduled for total hip or knee arthroplasty or hip fracture surgery

	Prophylactic dose/day
Unfractionated heparin	3 × 5,000 UI (sc)
Low-molecular-weight heparins	≥3,500 UI[a]
Fondaparinux	2.5 mg
Dabigatran	220 mg (first dose 110 mg)
	150 mg in elderly (first dose 75 mg)
Rivaroxaban	10 mg
Apixaban	2 × 2.5 mg
Vitamin k antagonists	Adjusted for INR target 2.5

[a]Dose depending on the LMWH considered

Table 9.2 Patients at risk of bleeding or who need special care for assessment for possible risk of bleeding

Congenital bleeding disorders (as hemophilia or von Willebrand's disease)
Acquired bleeding disorders (as liver insufficiency or creatinine clearance <30 mL/min)
Treatment with antiplatelet drugs (as clopidogrel, prasugrel, or aspirin)
Concurrent use of anticoagulant drugs (as warfarin or Coumadin with INR > 1.5 the day of surgery or any direct oral anticoagulant indicated by medical reasons)
Patient receiving chronically anti-inflammatory drugs
Personal or familiar history of bleeding episodes
Known prolonged or altered coagulation tests (INR or aPTT)
Thrombocytopenia (less than 75×10^9/L) or thrombocytopathy
Recent (<6 months) acute stroke
Lumbar puncture/epidural/spinal anesthesia within the previous 4 h or expected within the next 12 h
Uncontrolled systolic hypertension

Personal adaptation from Refs. [2, 4]

procedure, the availability of the drug in each country or hospital, the local recommendations, the common local or personal practice, etc. Table 9.1 shows the recommended daily dosage of each drug for thromboprophylaxis, and main characteristics are revised in other chapters of the book.

Due to the high risk of VTE in these kinds of patients, and the strong evidence that pharmacological prophylaxis reduces it [3], as key general recommendation, the main evidence is the administration of pharmacological thromboprophylaxis, which is mandatory if the thrombotic risk outweighs the bleeding one. In those patients with "too high" bleeding risk (Table 9.2) or those so-called fragile patients (body weight under 50 kg, mild renal insufficiency, aged more than 80 years, …), the use of mechanical devices could be the best option [2, 4], although they provide an inferior protection against VTE. Finally, the use of both methods (one drug plus one mechanical device) has been recently recommended to increase the efficacy of both when used separately [5].

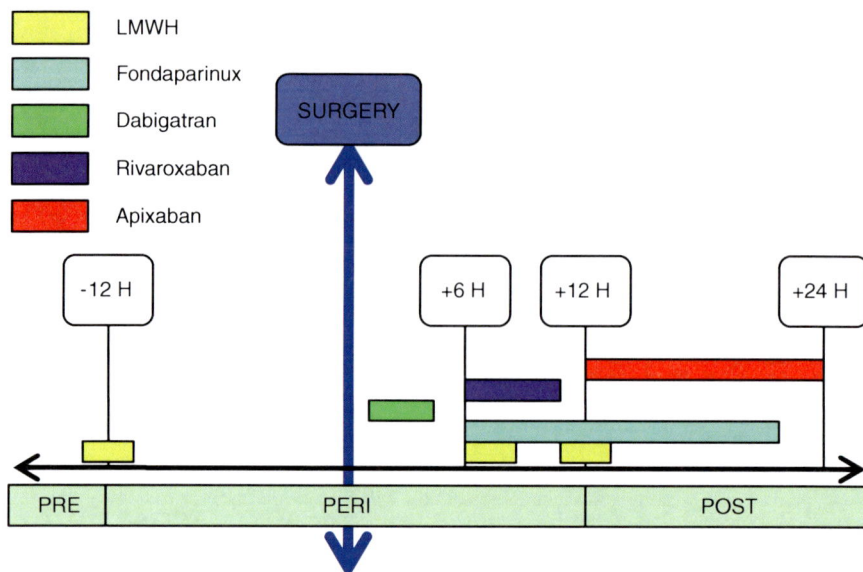

Fig. 9.1 Compilation for the administration of first dose of thromboprophylaxis in patients undergoing THA or TKA, in dependence of the chosen drug

Timing for the First Dose of Anticoagulant

Each drug used for thromboprophylaxis has its own "time to start" around surgery. In some cases, there is a consensus: for example, the first dose of fondaparinux must be given at least 6 h after the end of surgery or direct oral anticoagulants (rivaroxaban, apixaban, or dabigatran) must be started after surgery. Nevertheless, the consensus is not general when we speak about LMWH, and they are given in different protocols depending on the country and, mainly, on the clinical practice. In Fig. 9.1, we have summarized the accepted time for the administration of the first dose of anticoagulants for thromboprophylaxis in patients undergoing TKA or THA.

Related with LMWH, some controversies have issued from many years, and nowadays, there is no evidence to strongly recommend one or the other protocol. Some interesting concerns in this question have been developed as follows:

- Some years ago, Raskob and Hirsh discussed about the best moment to begin prophylaxis in major orthopedic surgery [6], and they concluded that it is not necessary to begin preoperatively in order to have good efficacy and that the initiation at 6 h postoperatively is effective without increasing major bleeding risk. They suggested that the initiation 12–24 h postoperatively can be less effective than initiation at 6 h, proposing that 6 h could be the threshold for early postoperative administration.
- Lassen conducted a post hoc analysis from some trials in which they have used enoxaparin for the comparison with new oral anticoagulants and fondaparinux.

He concluded that, despite the enhanced convenience and safety of delaying the first administration of enoxaparin to the postoperative period, this strategy may not be appropriate in terms of efficacy and that the administration firstly 12 h postoperatively would be a suboptimal protocol [7].

- The NICE guide shows no doubt in this question, and it states that the administration of first dose of LMWH should be done in the postoperative period, at 6–12 h after the end of surgery [4]. There is no recommendation for the beginning before surgery nor for the delay more than 12 h after the end of surgery.
- An observational study comparing the administration of the same dose of enoxaparin (40 mg) 12 h before knee surgery and 6–12 h after the end of it found no difference in terms of efficacy or safety [8]. The authors concluded that the postoperative beginning is an option which should be preferred if the patient is going to receive regional anesthesia or if the patient is admitted to the hospital the same day of the scheduled surgery.
- The French Society of Anesthesiology has updated the consensus document for the management of thromboprophylaxis in these patients, and they disagree with the suggestions of Lassen. When a LMWH is the drug chosen, the recommendation is to begin in the postoperative period [9]. The main reason for this recommendation is that they do not found any difference in terms of efficacy between the beginning in the preoperative or in the postoperative period, and they consider the postoperative beginning better because of the high use of neuraxial anesthesia in patients undergoing major orthopedic surgery. The FOTO study demonstrates that around three quarters of patients operated of TKA or THA received the first dose of LMWH in the postoperative period as clinical practice, avoiding (perhaps without really deep evidence) the preoperative dose [10].
- A recent multidisciplinary guide in Italy recognizes a great difficulty to recommend the beginning in the preoperative or in the postoperative period, and they do not find any agreement [2]. So, from this guideline, the recommendation is that thromboprophylaxis can be started either pre- or postoperatively, although they state that in some LMWH labels, it is only recommended to start 12 h before surgery and no words are found for the postoperatively start.
- Finally, in the last paper from the American College of Chest Physicians, it is recommended to avoid the administration between 4 h before surgery and 4 h after it, because the risk of bleeding complications linked to the administration in this time period is unacceptable [5]. They recommend to start 12 h before surgery or from 12 h after it. Both protocols should have similar effectiveness and safety, and they state no evidence of superiority of one over the other.

Main Recommendations for Total Hip Arthroplasty or Total Knee Arthroplasty

To offer the most recent and complete guide for thromboprophylaxis in patients undergoing THA or TKA, we have tried to mix up the recommendations from some articles that we consider of outstanding interest.

- Patients undergoing THA or TKA must receive thromboprophylaxis. The kind of drug, the best mechanical device to be used, and all the details related with the beginning and duration of thromboprophylaxis should be decided once the patient has been assessed on his/her personal circumstances and comorbidities.
- In patients undergoing THA or TKA, the preference is the administration of a pharmacological prophylaxis. The clinicians can choose between LMWH, fondaparinux, apixaban, dabigatran, and rivaroxaban, low dose of UFH, or adjusted dose of vitamin K antagonist (VKA). The aspirin has been rejected in most of guidelines [2–4, 9], but it has been included as one possibility for prophylaxis in last ACCP guidelines [5]. The personal opinion of the authors is that aspirin is not as efficacious as the other drugs proposed, and the low risk of bleeding related to the other drugs does not justify this recommendation.
- Between the pharmacological options for thromboprophylaxis in patients undergoing THA or TKA, the preference is not clear, but we can state next considerations.

  - The most widely drugs used all over the world are LMWH. They are efficacious and easy to use, they have demonstrated good safety profile, and the clinicians have huge experience with them. Probably, by these reasons, the last ACCP guidelines recommend "the use of LMWH in preference to the others agents recommended as alternatives" [5]. For the anesthesiologist, the administration of a LMWH as prophylaxis in patients undergoing THA or TKA has the advantage of the good, easy, and safe recommendations related with the performance of regional anesthesia [11].
  - New oral anticoagulants (apixaban, dabigatran, and rivaroxaban) are also very good options. In general, they are at least as efficacious as LMWH, and in some cases, they have better efficacy results in recent trials [12–14]. The associated risk of bleeding does not exceed the benefits reached with them, but in the so-called fragile patients, this question could be a limitation for its choice as the first option in prophylaxis. It is necessary to bear in mind the known advantages of the new oral anticoagulants, being the most important one the oral administration faced to the injection of LMWH or fondaparinux.
  - Fondaparinux is a very good drug, with a high efficacy (significantly more efficacious than LMWH in the prevention of venographic thrombotic events) and a slight increase in bleeding which does not exceed the benefits of the prevention of thrombotic events. The long half-life of fondaparinux could be a challenge for its administration in all patients as first option, due to its use in combination with postoperative analgesia through a peridural catheter, although it has been demonstrated that it is a safe combination having a skipped dose for the removal of the catheter [15].
  - Low dose of UFH or AVK is not the first option anywhere. Although their efficacy could place them close to LMWH, they are not as easy to use, and in the opinion of the authors, UFH and AVK should be placed in a second line of treatment possibilities.

- Mechanical prophylaxis is a good option for patients operated of arthroplasty. The main and most important kind of mechanical prophylaxis is postoperative mobilization: it must be started as soon as possible, and for bed rest patients, it is advisable to mobilize lower limbs, actively and/or passively. Between the other possibilities, intermittent pneumatic compression (IPC) is the best one and the first recommendation in recent guidelines over graduated compression stockings (GCS) [5]. Its use is effective alone or in combination with another method of prophylaxis in diminishing the risk of DVT in hospitalized patients. The main practical difficulty with IPC is patient compliance; also skin necrosis or discomfort can lead to poor compliance [3]. To be effective, it is necessary that the devices are used continuously while on bed rest in the postoperative period. So, in order to get better compliance, some clinicians prefer GCS over IPC. Finally, GCS alone give no enough protection in these patients, its use without pharmacological prophylaxis is recommended only in patients at risk of bleeding in which it is not possible to administrate an anticoagulant, and the IPC is not well tolerated.
- The duration of the administration of the thromboprophylaxis is also another point of discussion. The majority of VTE events occur after hospital discharge, so the evidence supporting the benefits for the prolongation of prophylaxis, once the patient is at home, is strong and makes it mandatory. But the cornerstone of this affirmation is how long this prolongation should be extended:

  - The minimum for prophylaxis is 10 days in all cases (THA and TKA) [2, 4], but this recommendation should be taken only as a "minimal time."
  - In patients undergoing TKA, it is suggested to prolong the prophylaxis until the day 35th, without a high level of evidence of benefit (2C) but with a low risk of associated bleeding. This practice is common between many orthopedists.
  - In patients undergoing THA, it is recommended to prolong the prophylaxis until the day 35th, without increase of the risk of bleeding and with an increase of efficacy against VTE. So the recommendation has a higher level of evidence (1B) in some guidelines [2, 9], although not in others [5].

Patients for Hip Fracture Surgery

The risk of VTE is very high in patients with HFS (between 50 and 70 % of patients with HFS could have a thrombotic event without prophylaxis [1, 4]), and it is higher if some personal factors are present: history of previous thrombotic event, more than 2 h of surgery, varicose veins, or more than 48 h of delay from the fracture to the time of surgery [9]. Moreover, the risk of these patients has the challenge of the age, because the vast majority of them are elderly patients.

We can summarize the main recommendations for thromboprophylaxis in patients with HFS as follows [2, 4, 5, 9]:

- LMWH and fondaparinux are two pharmacological options of first line of choice, over UFH or AVK. Fondaparinux is more efficacious than LMWH in the prevention of symptomatic thrombotic events (so-called in some references, venographic thrombi), but it associates a higher risk of bleeding, mainly in patients with moderate renal impairment [9]. Moreover, the choice of fondaparinux for thromboprophylaxis has the challenge of its no indication for preoperative administration, and the common delay of surgery found in many cases, which ranges from some hours to several days, mainly in cases of instability of the patient (cardiac compromise, diabetes decompensation, need for transfusions, and others).
- If the patient is going to be operated more than 12 h after his admission to the hospital, the first dose of anticoagulant must be given before surgery. In this case, the drug of choice is a LMWH, having in mind the safety window of 12 h between this administration and the optimal moment of surgery (not only to minimize the risk of bleeding associated to surgery but also the risk of spinal bleeding associated with a neuraxial anesthesia, widely performed in patients with HFS). After surgery, the clinician can change from the LMWH to fondaparinux if it is thought necessary due to a special thrombotic high risk associated.
- Aspirin has no indication for these patients as thromboprophylaxis, and its use as only agent cannot be recommended because the evidence suggests a poor efficacy. UFH is an option, but it has less efficacy than LMWH.
- New oral anticoagulants (apixaban, dabigatran, and rivaroxaban) have no indication in patients with HFS.
- Mechanical devices should be used in these patients, who should have a combined mechanical and pharmacological prophylaxis. IPC or GCS should be started at admission, choosing between them depending on the individual patient factors. The continuation of mechanical prophylaxis is recommended until the patient has no longer significantly reduced mobility.
- The duration of prophylaxis has to be extended for 28–35 days.

Conclusions

Patients undergoing a THA or TKA, or those with a HFS, have high risk to develop VTE, and it is mandatory to provide them thromboprophylaxis. But, nowadays, this sentence has many nonsolved controversies: the best drug (with the best risk-benefit balance); the best moment to begin; how the mechanical devices can aid in the prophylaxis both, alone, or in combination with the anticoagulants; which is the real role of aspirin and if it is honest to give it over other drug, which is the current and future role of new oral anticoagulants; how long it is necessary and optimal to extend the prophylaxis; etc.

All these topics have been revised in this chapter, and, briefly, recent guidelines have been compared, giving an overview of the best options for prophylaxis in these patients.

References

1. Geerts WH, Bergqvist D, Pineo GF, Heit JA, Samama CM, Lassen MR, et al. Prevention of venous thromboembolism. Chest. 2008;133:381S–453.
2. Della Rocca G, Biggi F, Gossi P, Imberti D, Landolfi R, Palareti G, et al. Italian intersociety consensus statement on antithrombotic prophylaxis in hip and knee replacement and in femoral neck fracture surgery. Minerva Anestesiol. 2011;77:1003–10.
3. Scottish Intercollegiate Guidelines Network (SIGN). Prevention and management of venous thromboembolism. Edinburgh: SIGN; 2010.
4. National Collaborating Centre for Acute and Chronic Conditions. Venous thromboembolism: reducing the risks. National Institute for Health and Clinical Excellence (NICE guide). London: National Institute for Health and Clinical Excellence (NICE); 2010.
5. Falck-Ytter Y, Francis CW, Johanson NA, Curley C, Dahl OE, Schulman S, et al. Prevention of VTE in orthopedic surgery patients: antithrombotic therapy and prevention of thrombosis, 9th ed: American College of Chest physicians evidence-based clinical practice guidelines. Chest. 2012;141:278S–325.
6. Raskob GE, Hirsh J. Controversies in timing of the first dose of anticoagulant prophylaxis against venous thromboembolism after major orthopedic surgery. Chest. 2003;124:379S–85.
7. Lassen MR. Is the preoperative administration of enoxaparin 40 mg necessary to optimally prevent the occurrence of venous thromboembolism after hip surgery? A subanalysis of two pooled randomized trials. J Thromb Haemost. 2009;7:889–91.
8. Llau JV. Clinical use of enoxaparin as thromboprophylaxis after total knee arthroplasty (TKA) in daily practice: an observational study: 6AP3-2. Eur J Anaesthesiol. 2011;28 Suppl 1:85.
9. Samama CM, Gafsou B, Jeandel T, Laporte J, Steib A, Marret E, et al. Prévention de la maladie thromboembolique veineuse postopératoire. Actualisation 2011. Texte court. Ann Fr Anesth Reanim. 2011;30:947–51.
10. Samama CM, Ravaud P, Parent F, et al. Epidemiology of venous thromboembolism after lower limb arthroplasty: the FOTO study. J Thromb Haemost. 2007;5:2360–7.
11. Gogarten W, Vandermeulen E, Van Aken H, Kozek S, Llau JV, Samama CM. Regional anaesthesia and antithrombotic agents: recommendations of the European Society of Anesthesiology. Eur J Anaesthesiol. 2010;27:999–1015.
12. Eriksson BI, Dahl OE, Rosencher N, Kurth AA, van Dijk GN, Frostick SP, et al. Oral dabigatran etexilate vs. subcutaneous enoxaparin for the prevention of venous thromboembolism after total knee replacement: the RE-MODEL randomized trial. J Thromb Haemost. 2007;5:2178–85.
13. Lassen MR, Raskob GE, Gallus A, Pineo G, Chen D, Hornick P. Apixaban versus enoxaparin for thromboprophylaxis after knee replacement (ADVANCE-2): a randomised double-blind trial. Lancet. 2010;375:807–15.
14. Lassen MR, Ageno W, Borris LC, Lieberman JR, Rosencher N, Bandel TJ, et al. Rivaroxaban versus enoxaparin for thromboprophylaxis after total knee arthroplasty. N Engl J Med. 2008;358:2776–86.
15. Singelyn FJ, Verheyen C, Piovella F, Van Aken HK, Rosencher N. The safety and efficacy of extended thromboprophylaxis with fondaparinux after major orthopedic surgery of the lower limb with or without a neuraxial or deep peripheral nerve catheter: the EXPERT study. Anesth Analg. 2007;105:1540–7.

Chapter 10
Thromboprophylaxis in Day Surgery: Knee Arthroscopy and Ligamentoplasty (Ligament Reconstruction)

James E. Muntz, Steven E. Flores, and Walter R. Lowe

Abstract This chapter discusses issues of non-large joint surgery, mainly knee arthroscopy and ligamentous knee injuries, and what to do in regard to prevention of venous thromboembolism in these patients. Events, if they occur, can be costly, associated with poor outcomes and, even in rare instances, death. The purpose of this chapter is to raise one's awareness of this complication as well as to assess risk stratification and decrease the occurrence of DVT in this orthopedic population.

Keywords Non-large joint surgery • DVT • Knee arthroscopy • Ligamentous knee injuries • Venous thromboembolism

Introduction

The occurrence and natural history of deep venous thrombosis (DVT) and pulmonary embolism (PE) after major orthopedic surgery has been elucidated throughout the medical and orthopedic literature over the last 30 years. It is now routine to provide thromboprophylaxis for essentially all total hip replacement, total knee replacement, and hip fracture patients. The same cannot be said for non-large joint

J.E. Muntz, M.D., FACP(✉)
Medicine and Orthopedics Departments, Baylor College of Medicine,
6550 Fannin Street, Suite 2339, Houston, TX 77030, USA

Memorial Hermann Sports Medicine Clinic,
Houston, TX, USA
e-mail: jmuntz@tmhs.org

S.E. Flores, M.D.
Department of Orthopedic Surgery,
University of Texas Health Science Center, Houston, TX, USA

W.R. Lowe, M.D.
Department of Orthopedic Surgery,
University of Texas Health Science Center, Houston, TX, USA

Memorial Hermann Sports Medicine Clinic,
Houston, TX, USA

J.V. Llau (ed.), *Thromboembolism in Orthopedic Surgery*,
DOI 10.1007/978-1-4471-4336-9_10, © Springer-Verlag London 2013

orthopedic surgery cases, specifically knee arthroscopy, including ligamentous injuries. We will discuss the particulars of preoperative thromboprophylaxis and postoperative management to avoid the pitfalls of deep vein thrombosis development as well as its known complications and morbidity.

Major orthopedic surgery of the hip and knee, specifically arthroplasty, carries a substantial risk for the occurrence of DVT that is described to be in the range of 40–50 % (per venographic trials) [1] when prophylaxis is not utilized. Patients who undergo arthroscopic procedures such as knee arthroscopy or ligamentous reconstruction are at risk for DVT but at a substantially lesser degree than large joint surgery patients. Despite this, it is important to recognize that arthroscopic knee surgery is the most commonly performed orthopedic procedure in the United States and worldwide [2]. These procedures are typically performed in young patients, often in day surgery settings, and one does not usually consider DVT a significant problem in this segment of the population. Because of these issues, the unexpected occurrence of a DVT makes the event even more catastrophic for both the patient and the physician performing the procedure.

Trials in Arthroscopic Procedures

An evaluation of prospective studies of knee arthroscopy without prophylaxis includes the early trial by Demers from Ontario, Canada [3]. The Canadian study revealed the surprising result of DVT occurrence (by venography) to be as high as 17.9 %. All clots that were found were either proximal or involving calf veins only. A total of 184 patients were included, none of whom developed a pulmonary embolism or suffered mortality [3]. A similar trial from Salt Lake City, Utah, revealed a much lower venographic rate of clot of just under 3 % [4]. Findings and data reviewed from these trials found that DVT occurrence was associated with tourniquet usage and prolonged operative time. An earlier prospective study published in the journal arthroscopy in 1995 involved only 85 patients with a clot rate identified at 3.5 % identified by compression ultrasound, all of which were clinically silent [5]. The venous clots in this trial involved calf veins that did not extend into the popliteal trifurcation, which would be considered a more ominous location for potential problems.

Ilahi et al. performed a meta-analysis on thromboprophylaxis in knee arthroscopy to provide data from a larger number of patients as all trials to date had included very small patient numbers. This meta-analysis included six trials and 684 patients who did not receive prophylaxis and underwent venography as an endpoint [6]. The incidence of overall DVT was 9.9 % with a proximal rate of 2.1 % by venography.

Just as DVT complications can occur from precipitating events such as large joint surgery and general and gynecologic procedures, clots that happen after arthroscopy can also have catastrophic outcomes with major morbidity and even mortality. Because these surgeries are performed in otherwise young, healthy patients, complications requiring an ICU admission, chronic leg swelling, and postthrombotic syndrome are unusual.

Several low molecular weight heparin trials involving thromboprophylaxis have been performed and are listed in Table 10.1. Michot et al. reported a relatively high risk of DVT in patients undergoing ambulatory arthroscopic knee surgery without

Table 10.1 Clinical trials of antithrombotics (low molecular weight heparin) for DVT prophylaxis in arthroscopy

Trial	Treatments	Patients	Trials design and methods
Dalteparin versus control			
Michot (2002) [7] n = 66/64 Follow-up: 30 days	Dalteparin 2,500 IU 60–120 min before procedure, followed 6 h after the end of the procedure by 2,500 IU (<70 kg) or 5,000 IU(>70 kg) versus no treatment	Patients requiring diagnostic or therapeutic arthroscopic knee surgery as outpatients; aged 18–80 years	Parallel groups open Switzerland
Enoxaparin versus control			
Canata (2003) [12] n = 18/18 Follow-up: 6 days	Enoxaparin sc daily (dose not specified) versus no treatment	ACL reconstruction for symptomatic ACL-deficient knees	Parallel groups Italy
Nadroparin versus control			
Kant (7 days) (2008) [2] n = 657/660 Follow-up: 3 months	Once-daily subcutaneous injection of LMWH (nadroparin, 3,800 anti-Xa IU) for 7 days versus full-length graduated compression stocking for 7 days	Patients undergoing knee arthroscopy	Parallel groups open (blinded assessment) Italy
Nadroparin 14 days versus control			
Kant (14 days) (2008) [2] n = 444/660 Follow-up: 3 months	Once-daily subcutaneous injection of LMWH (nadroparin, 3800 anti-Xa IU) for 14 days versus full-length graduated compression stocking for 7 days	Patients undergoing knee arthroscopy	Parallel groups open (blinded assessment) Italy
Reviparin versus control			
Wirth (2001) [8] n = 117/122 Follow-up: 7–10 days	Reviparin 1,750 anti Xa IU Sc once daily for 7–10 days versus no treatment	Elective knee arthroscopy	Parallel groups open (blinded assessment) Germany

More details on http://www.trialresultscenter.org/godirect.asp?q=150

Table 10.2 Main ACCP recommendations for thromboprophylaxis in patients undergoing day surgery in orthopedics [1]

For patient undergoing knee arthroscopy who do not have additional risk factors (for DVT), we suggest that clinicians not routinely use thromboprophylaxis other than early mobilization (Grade 2B)
For patients undergoing arthroscopy who have additional thromboembolic risk factors or following a complicated procedure, we recommend thromboprophylaxis with low molecular weight heparin (Grade 1B)

the use of thromboprophylaxis. The use of the low molecular weight heparin dalteparin reduced the risk of DVT. In those who were randomized to the prophylaxis group, the risk of lower extremity venographic DVT was 1.5 % as opposed to 15.6 % in the control group of patients who did not receive the prophylaxis (p value 0.004) [7]. In a similar situation, the use of the low molecular weight heparin, reviparin, had the effects of a relative risk reduction of venographic clot formation by 80 % compared to the placebo group [8]. In this rather small sample, it would seem that thromboprophylaxis did indeed help deter the development of clots.

Recommendations for Thromboprophylaxis

Due to the lack of data and evidence, it would be prudent to look at the arthroscopy population and individualize patients by risk factors, injury, expected immobilization, etc., and identify a way to better protect an individual from clot formation. At the same time, one must minimize the risk of bleeding in the acute postoperative period that could further complicate the patient's recovery.

The Eighth ACCP Chest Consensus Conference on Antithrombotic and Thrombolytic Therapy has reviewed the existing literature and has made recommendations on prophylaxis for arthroscopic surgery [1]. Their guidelines are shown in Table 10.2.

We would like to combine data from previous LMWH trials that showed promise for deep venous thrombosis prevention with thromboprophylaxis with ACCP guidelines and apply this to current practice. One can individualize cases that fall into group 2 of the ACCP recommendation (additional risk factors or complex surgery) and make reasonable recommendations for DVT prevention. A number of years ago, Muntz discussed risk stratification by the Caprini model and made recommendation for DVT prophylaxis in non-large joint surgery patients [9]. This particular Caprini risk model is noted in Table 10.3 and is self-explanatory. One can see that as the risk factors mount (total factor score), the risk of clot formation is likely to increase and a more extensive or a longer duration of thromboprophylaxis may be indicated.

It is important to recognize that all recommendations that exist through ACCP involve usage of LMWH. One might extrapolate from successful trials in large joint orthopedic surgery that newer drugs discussed in other chapters of this textbook might be available for use in an "off-label" fashion for prophylaxis.

Table 10.3 Deep vein thrombosis prophylaxis risk factor assessment

Date: _____

ASSESSMENT: Please check all pertinent factors (Each risk factor has value of 1 unless otherwise noted.)	
☐ Age 35 to 60 years (1 point)	☐ *Pregnancy, or postpartum < 1 month*
☐ Age 61 to 70 years (2 points)	☐ C/S or operative vaginal delivery
☐ Age over 70 years (3 points)	
☐ Documented history of DVT or P.E. (3 points)	☐ Uterine instrumentation
	☐ Multiple trauma
☐ Family History of DVT or P.E.	☐ Inflammatory bowel disease
☐ Leg swelling, ulcers, stasis, varicose veins	☐ Hyperhomocysteinemia
☐ History of pelvic or long bone fracture	☐ Inherited thrombophilia (3 points):
☐ Lower extremity arthroscopy in patients > 50 years of age	* Activated protein C resistance (factor
☐ History of, or anticipated bed confinement/immobilization > 12 hours	* Antithrombin III deficiency
☐ Confining air/ground travel > 4 hours within 1 week of admission)	* Plasminogen or plasminogen activator deficiency
	* Protein C or S deficiency
☐ Spinal cord injury with paralysis	* Dysfibrinogenemia
☐ Stroke with paralysis	* Prothrombin Gene variant
☐ Mitral Valve Prolapse	☐ Antiphospholipid antibodies or Lupus anticoagulant (3 points)
☐ MI/CHF	
☐ Obesity (greater than20% over IBW)	☐ Non-hemorrhagic myeloproliferative disorders including polycythemia vera
☐ Shock/Dehydration	☐ Hyper viscosity syndromes
☐ Infection	☐ Plasminogen deficiency
☐ General anesthesia > 2 hours	☐ Estrogen hormone replacement therapy
☐ Other _____	

RISK ASSIGNMENT CATEGORY			
Low Risk:		**High Risk**	
Score of 1 or less	Moderate Risk	Score of 3 or 4	Very High Risk
	Score of 2		Score of 5 or >
or	**or**	**or**	**or**
* Minor Surgery	* Major Surgery and	Age 40 years **and**	*Major surgery in patients > 40 years with any of the following:
	*Age > 40 years with no additional risk factors	*Major surgery *Myocardial infarction and additional risk factors	*History of venous thromboembolism *Hip fracture or total joint procedures of leg *Stroke/spinal cord injury *Visceral malignancy *Additional risk factors

(continued)

Table 10.3 (continued)

SUGGESTED REGIMENS FOR PROPHYLAXIS IN EACH RISK CATEGORY			
Low Risk	**Moderate Risk**	High Risk	**Very High Risk**
*early ambulation	*LDUH every 8-12 hours, or	*LDUH (5,000 u every 8 hours, and	LMWH <u>or</u>
			*Oral anticoagulation with target INR 2.0 −3.0 <u>or</u>
	*SCD, <u>or</u>	2 hour preop), <u>or</u>	
*consider elastic stockings			
	+/−elastic stocking	*SCD <u>or</u> LMWH	*SCD + heparin (LMWH or LDUH)

CONTRAINDICATIONS TO ANTICOAGULATION THERAPY:

Relative (Check if applicable)   Absolute (Check if applicable)

☐   ☐

   Cerebral hemorrhage at any time   *Active hemorrhage from wounds, drains, lesions*
   previously

☐ GI, GU bleed or stroke with in past 6 months   ☐ Heparin use in RITT

☐ Thrombocytopenia   ☐ Warfarin use in pregnancy

☐ Coagulopathy   ☐ Severe trauma to head, spinal cord or extremities with

☐ Active Intracranial lesions/neoplasms   hemorrhage within 4 weeks

☐ Proliferative retinopathy

☐ Vascular access/biopsy sites inaccessible to hemostatic control

Contraindication to anticoagulants: No _____ Yes _____ (if yes, explain: _____)

PLEASE CHECK THE MODALITY (IES) CHOSEN FROM THE LIST BELOW AND SIGN/DATE:

☐   ☐ Warfarin (Regimen: _____)
   Elastic stockings

☐ Sequential compression device (SCD)   ☐ Other   (Specify: _____)

☐ Elastic stockings plus SCD   ☐ No prophylaxis

☐ LMWH (Regimen: _____)   ☐ Suspected DVT, perform diagnostics

☐ Heparin (Regimen: _____)

Attention: Follow Anesthesia Protocol for Epidural patients

LDUH-low dose unfractionated heparin

DVT-deep vein thrombosis

PE-pulmonary embolus

HITT-heparin induced thrombocytopenial

Patient Label

SCD-sequential compression on device

Physician's Signature:

IBW-ideal body weight

There are surgery specific issues that are associated with increased bleeding and patient-specific characteristics associated with unacceptable, excessive bleeding. The agents used for prophylaxis (agent-specific risk) also have certain bleeding concerns. A meta-analysis by Leonardi et al. examined bleeding complications after pharmacologic prophylaxis in general surgery patients (small number of orthopedic patients included) and examined the occurrence of injection site hematomas, wound complications, and GI and GU bleeding, along with rates of discontinuation of prophylaxis secondary to bleeding. Minor complications, bruising (6.9 %), wound hematoma (5.7 %), and drain site bleeding (2.0 %) were most common. Major complications were infrequent, i.e., gastrointestinal (0.2 %) or retroperitoneal (<0.1 %) bleeding. A change in care was necessary in less than 3 % of patients and appeared to be reduced with lower-dose prophylaxis [10].

In addition to surgery and agent-specific issues, individual or patient-specific factors can be best delineated by review of bleeding data obtained from anticoagulation treatment trials. In general, patient factors that are felt to increase bleeding risks are increased age of the individual, other comorbid conditions such as hypertension (treated and untreated), ischemic stroke, heart disease, renal insufficiency [11], and liver disease. Additionally, if the patient is on antiplatelet medication (aspirin, clopidogrel, or COX_1 inhibitors), and additional pharmacologic agents are being considered, the risk of bleeding is likely to increase.

Sample Cases

The following are sample cases that take into consideration preop testing, drug administration, length of prophylaxis, etc. As mentioned earlier, it is equally important to minimize bleeding that can occur from surgery alone or surgery combined with pharmacologic agents as it is to prevent the formation of clots. The following cases are meant to explore real-life situations. There are different ways to handle these cases and not just one specific correct answer.

Case 1

A 25-year-old patient is injured in a ski mishap while in Colorado. The history and physical exam are unremarkable, and the patient is on no medication. Exam and MRI show a torn anterior cruciate ligament and no other serious injury. The patient is stabilized and flies home to Texas for scheduled repair in a couple of weeks. On the day of surgery, the patient's calf is noted to be swollen and sore per anesthesia, and the patient is sent for a venous Doppler ultrasound. The Doppler is read as positive for significant clot in the peroneal and posterior tibial veins:

1. Surgery is postponed and the patient then receives treatment dosage of low molecular weight heparin.
2. What if the patient was a 45-year-old female on hormone replacement therapy and her preoperative flight was from Colorado to London, England? Would one use thromboprophylaxis? According to ACCP 8th Consensus Conference, the patient has additional risk factors at time of arthroscopic surgery, namely, HRT, and possibly travel thrombosis should be considered.
3. What if the 25-year-old patient is noted to have had a preoperative PTT that is slightly prolonged? Further preop testing determines that the patient is positive for the lupus anticoagulant as the cause of prolongation of the PTT:

(a) Thromboprophylaxis in the perioperative period?
(b) Length and duration of prophylaxis … type of agent?
(c) Start time? Preop, post-op day zero, or postoperative day 1?
(d) Does one test family members for thrombophilia? (Lupus anticoagulant is an acquired and not congenital hypercoagulable state.)

Case 2

A college student injures his knee in an amateur neighborhood football game, sustaining a tear of the anterior cruciate ligament with associated damage to the posterior cruciate ligament. Initially, ice is used to prevent swelling, and the student does not seek medical care for 48 h. Swelling at that time is significant and an MRI is performed, confirming the initial diagnosis. Surgery will be delayed for 10–14 days until swelling resolves and range of motion returns:

1. Should DVT prophylaxis be utilized in the 10–14 day presurgical time period while the patient is immobile and awaiting surgery?
2. The patient receives 2 days of prophylactic low molecular weight heparin and notices marked increase in swelling, bleeding, and ecchymosis up and down the leg. The LMWH is stopped for 4–5 days or longer until hemostasis is no longer an issue.
3. Preop Doppler ultrasound if swelling increases off the anticoagulant to rule out any DVT.

Case 3

A 17-year-old male is scheduled to undergo ACL reconstruction using patellar tendon autograft and inside-out medial meniscus repair. His family has a history of clotting issues, one uncle with a history of DVT, and a sister with prior pulmonary embolism suspected to be hormone related. He would fall under "elevated risk of clot" with a "standard risk of bleeding." The decision to place patient on standard LMWH prophylaxis is made to begin on post-op day one.

Surgery is performed under tourniquet use without complications. The patient is seen on postoperative day one and found to have a large hemarthrosis causing significant pain and is subsequently aspirated. Medial wound and harvest sites are intact:

1. The decision to begin prophylaxis is delayed secondary to significant post-operative bleeding.
2. The patient is seen back on post-op day four and found to still have a significant, all be it smaller effusion with wounds continuing to heal.

3. Due to patient's classification as "elevated risk" and inability to adequately prophylax, the surgeon elects to proceed with a screening Doppler ultrasound at day 7 and 14 post-op to determine presence or absence of clot which wound potentially change management.

Table 10.4   Knee arthroscopy and ligamentoplasty recommendations [1]

Consideration	Duration of prophylaxis	Level of evidence
Decision to prophylax	7–10 days	Expert opinion
Immobility and non-weightbearing	Until risk is diminished (range of motion or weight-bearing restored)	Expert opinion
Current warfarin use	Restart warfarin post op	Expert opinion
Prior clot development after orthopedic surgery	Continue anticoagulation several weeks beyond time it took for prior clot to develop	Expert opinion
History of thrombophilia	>10 days	Expert opinion
Patient on antiplatelet meds for cardiac stent	Restart when hemostasis adequate	Grade 2C

From the above examples, it is evident that each clinical situation presents individualized challenges in determining the need for DVT prophylaxis, the consideration of bleeding risk, and the surgical timing decisions that are inherent within these clinical examples.

Duration of Prophylaxis

Although there is little published information on the prophylaxis of arthroscopy and ligamentous surgical patients, there is even less data available on duration of thromboprophylaxis.

How is one to approach this subject other than to extract data on duration of prophylaxis from orthopedic surgery in general? Table 10.4 is presented to help practitioners develop a plan in regard to the initiation and length of treatment. It should be noted that since no established protocol exists, the following recommendations are based on a combination of the information presented in this chapter and expert opinion.

Conclusion

Although the data is sparse and the levels of recommendations for DVT assessment and drug administration for arthroscopic and ligamentous knee surgeries are at low levels of evidence, this chapter outlines the available literature on this topic and aids an individual surgeon or medical care provider in better assessing patients for risk of DVT without producing an unacceptable risk to bleeding.

One should assess risk of DVT occurrence; individually assess bleeding concerns by patient, surgery, and agent-specific characteristics; and then determine if the benefits of treatment outweigh the risks. Drugs, both available on the market, and newer drugs, such as thrombin inhibitors and anti-Xa drugs, can provide treatment options. One must remember that cost, ease of administration, and compliance need to be considered to assist in obtaining successful surgical outcomes and decrease postoperative morbidity.

References

1. Geerts WH, Bergqvist D, Pineo GF, et al. Prevention of venous thromboembolism: the eighth ACCP conference on antithrombotic and thrombolytic therapy. Chest J. 2008;133(6): 381S–453S.
2. Camporese G, Bernardl E, Prandoni P, et al. Low-molecular-weight heparin versus compression stockings for thromboprophylaxis after knee arthroscopy: a randomized trial. Ann Intern Med. 2008;149(2):73–82.
3. Demers C, Marcoux S, Ginsberg JS, et al. Incidence of venographically proved deep vein thrombosis after knee arthroscopy. Arch Intern Med. 1998;158(1):47–50.
4. Jaureguito JW, Greenwald AE, Wilcox JF, et al. The incidence of deep venous thrombosis after arthroscopic knee surgery. Am J Sports Med. 1999;27(6):707–10.
5. Williams JS, Hulstyn MJ, Fadale PD, et al. Incidence of deep vein thrombosis after arthroscopic knee surgery: a prospective study. Arthroscopy. 1995;11(6):701–5.
6. Ilahi OA, Reddy J, Ahmad I. Deep venous thrombosis after knee arthroscopy: a meta-analysis. Arthroscopy. 2005;21(6):727–30.
7. Michot M, Conen D, Holtz D, et al. Prevention of deep-vein thrombosis in ambulatory arthroscopic knee surgery: a randomized trial of prophylaxis with low-molecular weight heparin. Arthroscopy. 2002;18(3):257–63.
8. Wirth T, Schneider B, Misselwitz F, et al. Prevention of venous thromboembolism after knee arthroscopy with low-molecular weight heparin (reviparin): results of a randomized controlled trial. Arthroscopy. 2001;17(4):393–9.
9. Muntz JE. The risk of venous thromboembolism in non-large joint surgeries. Orthopedics. 2003;26(2 Suppl):s237–42.
10. Leonardi MJ, McGory ML, Ko CY. The rate of bleeding complications after pharmacologic deep venous thrombosis prophylaxis: a systematic review of 33 randomized controlled trials. Arch Surg. 2006;141(8):790-7; discussion 797-9.
11. Van der Meer FJ, Rosendaal FR, Van den Broucke JP, et al. Bleeding complications in oral anticoagulant therapy. An analysis of risk factors. Arch Intern Med. 1993;153(13):1557–62.
12. Canata GL, Chiey A. Prevention of venous thromboembolism after ACL reconstruction: a prospective, randomized study. International Society of Arthroscopy, Knee Surgery and Orthopaedic Sports Medicine, 2003; Poster 71-2003.

Chapter 11
Thromboprophylaxis in Special Patients: Multiple Trauma, Head Trauma, and Spine Surgery

Maria J. Colomina, Lidia Mora, and Esther Ciércoles

Abstract There is a significant clinical association between a traumatic event and the development of venous thromboembolism (VTE). In this chapter, we are reviewing VTE in patients with multiple trauma, head trauma, or acute spinal cord injury and in those undergoing spine surgery: to gain knowledge about the incidence of thromboembolic events in these specific conditions, to identify patients at high risk for this complication, to establish whether there is a safe period during which anticoagulant therapy can be delayed, to determine the risk of bleeding according to the type of drug given, and to provide a basis upon which appropriate thromboprophylactic protocols can be worked out and implemented.

In most trauma patients, thromboprophylaxis with LMWH can be started at 48 h, and in patients with active bleeding, mechanical compression should be considered, despite its limited effectiveness, until the risk of hemorrhage has decreased. In elective spinal surgery, the thromboembolic risk is relatively low, and the use of mechanical devices as primary prophylaxis seems reasonable. The currently available evidence does not suffice to support or negate the use of anticoagulant agents in this surgery, but it does exclude routine application, based on the low risk of fatal pulmonary embolism. These agents are, however, appropriate for patients with acute spinal cord injury, who require lengthy bed rest. There is not enough data to justify routine screening with ultrasound or venography in all these cases. Multimodal treatment (mechanical and pharmacological) that guarantees optimal thromboprophylaxis in this type of patient currently implies a rational, multidisciplinary decision, supported by evidence-based medicine.

Keywords Thromboprophylaxis • Trauma patient • Spine surgery • Head trauma Mechanical devices • Anticoagulant therapy

M.J. Colomina, M.D., Ph.D. (✉) • L. Mora, M.D. • E. Ciércoles, M.D.
Anaesthesia Department, Hospital Universitario Vall d'Hebron,
Pssg. Vall d'Hebron 119–129, 08035 Barcelona, Spain
e-mail: mjcolomi@vhebron.net; mjcolomina@gmail.com

J.V. Llau (ed.), *Thromboembolism in Orthopedic Surgery*,
DOI 10.1007/978-1-4471-4336-9_11, © Springer-Verlag London 2013

Introduction

There are several important reasons for reviewing venous thromboembolism (VTE), a term encompassing deep venous thrombosis (DVT) and pulmonary embolism (PE), in patients with multiple trauma, head trauma, or acute spinal cord injury and in those undergoing spine surgery: to gain knowledge about the incidence of thromboembolic events in these specific conditions, to identify patients at high risk for this complication, to establish whether there is a safe period during which anticoagulant therapy can be delayed, to determine the risk of bleeding according to the type of drug given, and to provide a basis upon which appropriate thromboprophylactic protocols can be designed.

Various studies have focused on determining measures to prevent VTE in trauma and spine surgery patients, but they show a lack of homogeneity and important methodological limitations [1–7]. These include bias in patient selection and randomization, statistical weakness due to a small sample size, and missing information required to extrapolate the results, such as the population characteristics (demographic data, associated risk factors, type and location of the injury and related symptoms, severity scale scores), examination methods used (venography, Doppler ultrasound, computed tomography [CT] with angiography), duration and type of prophylaxis, duration of immobilization and hospitalization, and blood transfusion requirements. There are also shortcomings in proper stratification of the population according to age, treatment, proximal or distal DVT, presence of PE, and other factors.

Venous Thromboembolism in Multiple Trauma and Head Trauma Patients

There is a significant clinical association between a traumatic event and the development of VTE. The incidence of this complication ranges from 7 to 58 % depending on the demographic characteristics of the patients, the nature of the lesions implicated, the diagnostic methods used, and the type of prophylaxis administered [8]. In the absence of prophylactic measures, patients with severe trauma have a higher risk (>50 %) of developing VTE than other hospitalized patients. In a large study of patients with severe multiple trauma, DVT was documented on contrast venography performed at 1–3 weeks of hospitalization in 58 % of patients who did not receive thromboembolic prophylaxis and in 27 % of those who received routine treatment [9].

Pulmonary embolism is one of the causes of late mortality in multiple trauma patients and contributes substantially to the associated morbidity. It is the third cause of death in those that survive the first day following injury [7]. Approximately, 1 % of these patients present a proven, symptomatic episode of PE.

Although DVT mainly occurs in patients with severe systemic involvement, a recent case-control study has shown an increased risk even in patients with less severe trauma, the event occurring within 4 weeks after the accident. The association between lower limb fractures and VTE has been recognized since 1934, when McCartney observed a relationship between these fractures and later death due to PE [10].

The incidence of thromboembolism in head trauma, which ranges from 0.38 to 54 % [11], is difficult to precisely establish because of the variability of the populations studied and the methods used. In a retrospective study including 280 trauma patients with a high thrombotic risk, the incidence of VTE in the subgroup with traumatic head injury was 5 % [11]. In another retrospective study evaluating the incidence of PE in 94,044 patients hospitalized in an American trauma center between 1992 and 1996 [12], the VTE incidence was 0.38 % among 47,996 patients with head trauma, a figure significantly lower than that seen in the group without head injury (0.27 %). A Glasgow Coma Scale (GCS) score of ≤8 in head trauma patients increased the incidence of PE to 0.68 %. It is difficult to derive conclusions from these findings because the methods used for antithrombotic prophylaxis were not reported.

Pathophysiology of Venous Thromboembolism in Multiple Trauma and Head Trauma Patients

Venous stasis, endothelial injury, and hypercoagulability (Virchow's triad) are the main factors that intervene in the pathogenesis of a posttrauma prothrombotic state, which is also favored by the tendency toward a reduction in cytokines that inhibit systemic fibrinolysis [13]. In VTE, venous stasis allows activated coagulation factors to accumulate at sites prone to thrombosis (injured areas). Venous endothelial changes seem to be important only in the areas associated with direct trauma, but intimal injury and endothelial dysfunction may be key triggering mechanisms of hypercoagulability. The normally antithrombogenic endothelium becomes prothrombotic, and this is followed by greater platelet adhesion, activation of the procoagulant system, and increased thrombin generation. The factors contributing to the high incidence of VTE in trauma patients are, therefore, the systemic hypercoagulability state, immobilization due to skeletal traction for fractures, the patient's critical condition, and the presence of multiple venous lesions [14].

Apart from patients with related risk factors (malignant disease, venous insufficiency, cardiorespiratory failure), DVT seems to be more common in young patients who have no associated disease. In a study of 101 severe trauma patients, Meissner et al. reported a DVT rate of 27.7 % and a PE rate of 1.9 % [15]. VTE was significantly more common in obese patients older than 40 years, with prolonged immobilization lasting more than 3 days, pelvic injury, and fractures of the long bones. Nonetheless, on multivariate analysis, only obesity and immobilization were independent predictive factors of PE. Some authors also consider blood transfusion a risk factor for thromboembolism [15]. Few methodologically robust studies have been able to elucidate other predictive factors of risk apart from fracture of the long bones and pelvic trauma. The Injury Severity Score (ISS) results and use of multiple transfusions are not considered important [16].

A recent study has suggested that head trauma, in itself, is an independent risk factor for developing VTE, based on the following considerations: long immobilization period because of coma, presence of associated lesions in the case of multiple trauma, delays in thromboembolic prophylaxis when intracranial hemorrhage is diagnosed, concern about the consequences of increased volume, and hypercoagulability status resulting from platelet activation, massive release of tissue factor, and elevated levels of other procoagulants, such as von Willebrand factor [11].

Severe head trauma was considered one of the six independent risk factors for DVT in a recent analysis of 450,375 trauma patients registered in the American College of Surgeons National Trauma Data Bank [9]. Other risk factors were age >40 years, severe pelvic or lower limb fracture, vertebral fracture with complete spinal cord injury, >3 days on mechanical ventilation, venous lesions, episode of shock at hospitalization, and undergoing major surgery. The recommendations derived from this study to assess VTE risk in trauma patients are based on two major risk factors, the presence of vertebral fractures and spinal cord lesion. Advanced age is an additional risk factor, but it is not clear at what age risk significantly increases.

Bleeding Risk and Thromboprophylaxis in Trauma and Head Trauma Patients

The controversy regarding when to start thromboprophylaxis is based on the premise that any agent affecting hemostasis has hemorrhagic potential that can lead to increased bleeding in injured tissue. Uncontrolled bleeding accounts for 30–40 % of trauma-related mortality and is the main preventable cause of death in hospitalized multiple trauma patients [8]. Cessation of bleeding following injury depends on immediate induction of a prothrombotic state, and this becomes one end point in ongoing treatment whose main objective is survival of the patient. A randomized, placebo-controlled double-blind trial (CRASH 2) performed in 20,211 trauma patients concluded that tranexamic acid significantly reduces the overall mortality and mortality related to severe blood loss in this population [17].

The obvious disadvantage of inducing a prothrombotic state is the development of thrombotic complications. Prevention of VTE without interrupting the hemostatic capacity of injured vessels is a considerable challenge, and currently, definitive treatment options are not available. Nor has the optimal thromboprophylaxis method been conclusively defined in randomized controlled trials [13]. Often, appropriate prophylaxis is not prescribed in patients with neurotraumatic injury and ICH, spinal cord or solid-organ injury, or complex pelvic fractures because of concern about an increased risk of bleeding. Despite the available clinical practice recommendations, thromboprophylaxis is underused in 40–60 % of hospitalized patients with a risk of VTE.

Thromboprophylaxis Methods in Multiple Trauma and Head Trauma Patients

Few studies have focused on analyzing the usefulness of different types of thrombo-prophylaxis in the trauma population, and there are no treatment guidelines that define the optimal time to start this therapy or its duration. In 2006, Velmahos pub-lished two editorials on this subject [1, 2] and described the inconsistencies of the results provided by research with methodological problems.

Currently, there are two main methods of thromboprophylaxis: mechanical methods, including graduated compression stockings and intermittent pneumatic compression (IPC) devices, and pharmacologic methods, mainly heparin administration.

Mechanical Compression

The efficacy of mechanical thromboprophylaxis methods in hospitalized patients has been amply documented. Their main advantages are the absence of associated bleeding risk, ease of use, and relatively low cost [13]. The role of IPC devices has also been validated in trauma patients. IPC acts by decreasing venous stasis, and it has an indirect enhancing effect on fibrinolysis by shortening the euglobulin lysis time. In a prospective study, Knudson et al. compared IPC use with nonfractionated heparin administration and no prophylaxis [18]. The study showed that mechanical measures did not provide protection against VTE in multiple trauma patients with the exception of the subgroup of neurotrauma patients, in which IPC was significantly more effective than no prophylaxis for this purpose. In contrast, Gersin et al. evalu-ated the incidence of DVT in 32 patients with severe head trauma (GCS < 8) in a nonrandomized prospective study. Fourteen patients were treated with IPC, and 18 could not benefit from this measure because they presented fractures of the lower limbs. In the group treated with IPC, 4 (28 %) patients developed PE, and none presented DVT. In the group that did not receive prophylaxis, there were two cases of PE and two of DVT. Although the sample studied was small, the results obtained revived the existing debate about the efficacy of IPC in these patients [19]. Some of the most notable complications related to IPC use include peroneal nerve paralysis, compartmental syndrome, and skin necrosis.

In patients with severe head injury, another potential drawback to IPC is the pos-sibility of increasing intracranial pressure. This issue was investigated by Davidson et al., who evaluated 24 patients with severe head trauma (GCS ≤ 6) and calculated the intracranial pressure and cerebral perfusion pressure at 0, 10, 20, and 30 min of IPC application. The authors found no significant increase in intracranial pressure or cerebral perfusion pressure and concluded that IPC could be safely used in head trauma [20].

Despite its limitations, IPC is recommended in all patients undergoing neurosurgery because it is safe, well tolerated, can be used in combination with other methods, and has shown some efficacy in decreasing the incidence of VTE. In addition, it could be advantageous in patients with head injury and pathological bleeding, in whom heparin is contraindicated [7].

When mechanical devices are used alone, the protection achieved is not optimal. An analysis of five studies in patients hospitalized in critical care areas, comparing a mechanical thromboprophylaxis method with no prophylaxis, reported a 57 % reduction in the incidence of DVT. However, in patients treated exclusively with graduated compression stockings, venography demonstrated DVT in 32 % of cases, including proximal DVT in 13 % and clinically symptomatic phlebitis in 6 % [13]. Another study suggested that there is a statistically significant difference in the incidence of DVT in patients using bilateral IPC, although it remained unclear whether bilateral compression was indeed applied in all patients [21].

Currently, the use of IPC devices is recommended in patients with traumatic injury to the upper limbs, head, and chest. Additional study is needed to determine whether there is a difference between unilateral and bilateral IPC use, as an important variable affecting the incidence of thromboembolic events [22].

Heparin

Although low molecular weight heparin (LMWH) has been one of the most highly effective and widely used thromboprophylaxis modalities, the optimal administration approaches for this agent in trauma patients remain uncertain. Progress has been made in establishing the regimens for complex pelvic fractures, lower limb lesions that require lengthy periods of immobilization, and head trauma. Unfortunately, these do not encompass multiple trauma patients, and therefore, the current treatment recommendations continue to be extrapolations from other populations [2].

Unfractionated Heparin

The use of unfractionated heparin (UFH) remains unresolved. Recommendations from the United States suggest that in trauma cases in which bleeding can aggravate existing lesions (e.g., ICH, SCI, intraocular hemorrhage, pelvic trauma, severe lower limb trauma, and hematomas in unoperated intra-abdominal solid organs), administration of UFH thromboprophylaxis is not safe and should only be used within multidisciplinary protocols based on consensus [8, 16]. In a meta-analysis from the Agency for Healthcare Research and Quality, Velmahos et al. reviewed all randomized controlled clinical trials focusing on the use or not of UFH in trauma. The authors reported that UFH shows some efficacy in preventing

VTE in severe trauma, but most of the studies analyzed had methodological deficiencies, which suggested the possibility of statistical errors and detracted from the results [1].

Low Molecular Weight Heparin

LMWH has been recommended as thromboprophylaxis in patients with multiple injuries and has shown efficacy in reducing DVT and PE rates [7, 13, 14, 18]. The advantages of its use in comparison with other types of heparins include easy administration, higher efficacy and specificity relative to UFH (produces less bleeding at equivalent antithrombotic doses in relation to the effect on platelet function and vascular patency), and the fact that there is no need for specific biochemical monitoring [13]. In some studies, the use of enoxaparin is supported in trauma patients with a moderate or high risk of DVT and moderate risk of bleeding, and it is recommended as standard thromboprophylactic treatment, particularly in patients with complex pelvic fractures and lower limb injury [16].

Although subcutaneous administration of enoxaparin daily is safe and effective, some clinicians are reluctant to prescribe any thromboprophylactics, mainly in patients with solid-organ injury that have been treated conservatively [7]. In a retrospective study evaluating the percentage of bleeds in patients with spleen injury, no differences were found in transfusion or surgery requirements in patients receiving LMWH at 48 h following hospitalization compared to those given LMWH later [23]. These results were partially confirmed in a small prospective study evaluating treatment of spleen lesions, in which the need for surgical splenectomy because of conservative treatment failure coincided with administration of high LMWH doses at 12-h intervals [8].

In the absence of thromboprophylaxis or when the start of prophylaxis is delayed (>7 days), the VTE rate in head trauma patients is 20–25 % [11], and when prophylactic LMWH is administered 24 h following head injury, the VTE rate is between 0 and 4 % [24]. Reiff et al. demonstrated that the risk of DVT in head trauma increases according to the time interval during which prophylaxis is delayed, with a risk of 3.6 % when LMWH is given in the first 24 h, 4.5 % at 24–48 h, and 15.4 % after 48 h [25].

The low incidence of VTE reported in other studies may be due to the fact that most of the patients included were diagnosed and treated promptly. Nonetheless, this premise must take into account the potential risk of worsening an underlying ICH. In fact, early (<48 h) LMWH administration in patients with head injury seems to be associated with a higher risk of ICH progression [22, 24].

Because the majority of related studies are retrospective, the Brain Trauma Foundation guidelines [26] recommend LMWH or UFH for VTE prophylaxis in head trauma patients but also admit that there is a risk of increased ICH and that the available data do not suffice to recommend a specific agent, dose, or treatment duration. In most studies, the severity of the brain lesion is not specified, and authors encourage mechanical measures as first-line therapy while contraindicating LMWH in cases of active bleeding or an increase in intracranial hematomas until surgical evacuation has been performed and correct hemostasis confirmed [27].

Patients with severe head trauma and no evidence of a mass effect lesion (Marshall grade 1–4) should receive LMWH prophylaxis as soon as active bleeding at other locations is controlled; computed tomography (CT) study has been carried out at 12–24 h following the event, and no intracranial hematomas are documented [11].

With regard to head trauma with ICH, additional studies are needed to recommend LMWH thromboprophylaxis. In the cohort study by Norwood et al., 177 patients hospitalized with a documented diagnosis of ICH (95 with Marshall grade 2 lesions) were treated with enoxaparin 30 mg every 12 h, started at 24 h following admittance. ICH progression was visualized on CT in only 4 % of unoperated patients and 9 % of patients treated with craniotomy following the start of enoxaparin [28]. Based on these findings, a protocol change was considered, in which enoxaparin would be discontinued until 24 h following completion of the surgical procedure and restarted at 48–72 h to reduce VTE rates and ICH expansion.

Differences Between Different LMWHs

Various studies have focused on comparing enoxaparin versus dalteparin use in patients with head trauma and in those with spinal cord injury and traumatic bone lesions. A prospective study in 743 trauma patients with a high risk of DVT evaluated administration of a single daily dose of sodium dalteparin associated with IPC initiated in the first 36 h following hospitalization, after patients were hemodynamically stable and showed no evidence of active bleeding. The regimen was continued over the entire hospital stay, even when surgery or other invasive procedures were required, and it proved to be a safe option for thromboprophylaxis. There were no deaths attributable to bleeding complications following the start of treatment, transfusion requirements (3 %) were similar to reported values from other studies, and the incidence of PE (1–2 %) was considered reasonable in these patients. After adopting a protocol of continuous prophylaxis with daily LMWH administration, treatment compliance rates increased to 74 %. The authors considered this an important improvement in comparison to previous observations (33 %) [11, 24]. The most important conclusion was that there were no differences in VTE rates between patients treated with dalteparin or enoxaparin [11].

Adverse Effects of Heparin Treatment

Heparin-induced thrombocytopenia is a potentially fatal side effect of UFH administration (3–5 %) and less commonly of LMWH (0–0.9 %) [8]. In patients receiving these agents, platelet counts should be periodically monitored since the start of treatment. When thrombocytopenia is diagnosed, heparin administration should be interrupted, and an alternative treatment started. If possible, it should be a fast-acting one such as fondaparinux, a direct thrombin inhibitor because the risk of thrombosis in patients with induced thrombocytopenia is 30 times greater than in the general population [13, 23].

Bleeding complications are the most serious incidents recorded in studies reviewing heparin use, and they are particularly important in patients with intra-abdominal lesions treated conservatively and in those with head injury and ICH. Another important factor is to determine the start of prophylaxis according to the patient's hemodynamic stability. These two premises should be considered when deciding whether mechanical or pharmacological prophylaxis should be the first-line treatment in patients with multiple trauma [11, 16].

New Anticoagulant Treatments

Thromboprophylaxis with the new oral anticoagulants can provide the advantages of heparin and antivitamin K (AVK), with similar safety levels. The direct factor Xa inhibitor, rivaroxaban, has demonstrated a safety profile similar to enoxaparin in terms of bleeding risk. Furthermore, it is administered orally, and only one dose daily is needed, factors that can contribute to improving treatment compliance. Another oral treatment option is dabigatran etexilate, a direct thrombin inhibitor, which has demonstrated efficacy and safety similar to enoxaparin.

To date, there is no research on the use of these new drugs in multiple trauma patients, although they show promise as future options because of their potential efficacy, safety, and ease of administration [13].

Inferior Vena Cava Filter

Vena cava interruption is a prophylactic method to prevent PE that can be used in patients with severe trauma, active bleeding, head injury, spinal cord lesions, or ocular trauma and in those who are not candidates for other treatments because of a high probability of bleeding. It is also recommended in patients with a high thromboembolic risk, including those with neoplastic disease, hypercoagulability status, a history of thromboembolism, or spinal surgery using a combined anterior and posterior approach, an intervention involving five or more vertebrae, or anesthesia lasting more than 8 h. Other additional risk factors are an active smoking habit, obesity, oral contraceptive or hormone therapy use, substantial manipulation of the abdominal musculature or iliocaval area, and immobilization in bed for more than 2 weeks [4, 5, 8, 29, 30].

A comparative study was carried out in a prospective cohort of 39 high-risk patients who underwent vena cava filter implantation following spinal reconstruction and a historical control group of 122 patients who had undergone the same surgical procedure but without any type of prophylaxis [29]. Symptomatic PE was not diagnosed in any patient with filter implantation, compared to 13 % of patients with clinical signs of PE in the control group. This and other similar studies have provided the rationale for indicating placement of inferior vena cava

(IVC) filters to decrease the risk of PE only in very high-risk patients. Their use can also be considered in patients with spinal cord injury (SCI) receiving suboptimal prophylaxis but taking onto account that the risk of major complications derived from the implantation of the filter will be at least similar to the risk of developing a massive pulmonary embolism without the device. It has been estimated that if IVC filters are effective, they would need to be placed in 50 SCI patients receiving thromboprophylaxis to prevent one nonfatal PE at a cost of $250,000 [7].

Although IVC filters provide protection against PE, they expose the patient to a series of risks that should be considered: transferal of the patient to a specialized area, use of iodinated contrast material, possible vascular wall perforation, and migration of the filter to the right heart chambers or suprarenal vessels. Therefore, the use of these devices requires a consensus evaluation. The only absolute contraindications to IVC filters are IVC thrombosis and inability to access this vessel. In patients medically treated for DVT who have not received an IVC filter, the reported incidence of recurrent DVT at 5 years' follow-up is 13–24.6 %, which is very similar to the documented rates in patients with a filter [13].

Venous Thromboembolism in Spine Surgery Patients

There are no universally accepted guidelines recommending a specific protocol for VTE prevention in patients undergoing spine surgery. Several prophylactic methods have been used, but none have proven to be superior to the others. Furthermore, it is difficult to determine the incidence of postoperative VTE in this type of surgery. Studies that have documented DVT or PE vary with regard to the type of procedure and diagnostic methods used (physical examination, Doppler ultrasound, venography). A low incidence of DVT is expected in otherwise healthy patients who undergo only physical examination after short procedures that are not highly aggressive and a high incidence in patients with thromboembolic risk factors who undergo venography examination following major interventions. It has been observed that the postoperative incidence of DVT in spine surgery patients is underestimated when the diagnosis is based only on clinical examination. Nonetheless, the available evidence does not to suffice to justify routine postoperative screening with Doppler ultrasound or venography. In contrast to other orthopedic interventions, in spine surgery, there is no manipulation of the limbs, where thrombosis usually originates. When prophylactic pharmacological therapy is contemplated in these patients, it is important to assess the patient's risk of developing a symptomatic postoperative epidural hematoma, which could lead to secondary neurological deficits that imply a delay in patient mobilization and other comorbidities considered to be preventable complications, and weigh this risk against the benefits of VTE prevention [5, 6].

In a systematic review including 25 articles [30], the risk of DVT in spine surgery patients ranged from 0.3–31 %, with considerable variation depending on the population examined and the evaluation methods used. The overall incidence was 2.1 %, and incidence was seen to be influenced by the prophylaxis method used: no prophylaxis, 2.7 %; graduated compression stockings, 2.7 %; IPC, 4.6 %; compression stockings plus IPC 1.3 %; pharmacologic agents 0.6 %; and IVC filters with or without another prophylaxis method 22 %. Incidence was also influenced by the primary diagnostic follow-up method, with values of 1 % (clinical diagnosis), 3.7 % (Doppler ultrasound), and 12.3 % (venography). It is not possible to determine which method is the most cost-effective and has the greatest impact on survival based on the findings from this study. It did not clarify whether the presence of an asymptomatic DVT has an evident clinical impact or consider the cost-benefit risk of treating this condition. In this same review, the incidence of PE according to the prophylactic method used was as follows: overall 0.3 %, without prophylaxis 0.2 %, with graduated compression stockings or thigh-length compression stockings 0.6 %, IPC 1.1 %, IPC plus thigh-length stockings 1 %, pharmacological agents plus mechanical method 0.3 %, and IVC filter plus mechanical method 1 %. The incidence of DVT and PE based on the type of spine surgery was 3.4 and 0.1 %, respectively, following lumbar surgery and 1.1 and 1.2 % following major reconstructive surgery. In vertebral trauma, excluding SCI, the incidence of DVT/PE was 1.7/0.9 % and in tumor pathology, 1.2/0.7 %.

In another systematic review of 29 articles [6], the risk of thromboembolism determined in patients who did not receive pharmacological prophylaxis was slightly superior in corrective spinal surgery for deformity (DVT 5.3 %, range 2–14 %; PE 2.7 %, range 0–7.6 %) and in surgery for spinal trauma (DVT 6 %, range 0–19 %; PE 2 %, range 0–2.9 %) than in procedures for degenerative spinal disease (DVT 2.3 %, range 0–9 %; PE 0.4 %, range 0–1.5 %). Fatal pulmonary embolism was rare. In patients receiving pharmacological thromboprophylaxis, the DVT rate was 0–4.6 %, and the PE rate 0–2.2 %. Bleeding complications were uncommon when anticoagulation was used. The risk of severe hemorrhage ranged from 0 to 4.3 %, depending on the agent. Among the total of 2,507 patients reviewed, postoperative spinal hematoma was recorded in only ten cases [6]. As to the use of antiplatelet therapy, only one small study was found on this subject, in which no cases of bleeding were documented following ketorolac use. The authors of the review concluded that venous thromboembolism is uncommon following elective spine surgery. Nonetheless, it is likely that the true incidence of VTE was underestimated because of the sensitivity of the tests used (<100 %) and because some episodes may have presented after the examination was performed. Furthermore, various confounding variables may have masked important factors associated with DVT risk and affected the evaluation of thromboprophylaxis safety. Patients with vertebral trauma are at an increased risk of thromboembolic events and should be treated with pharmacologic agents, although the time interval during which anticoagulant administration can be safely delayed remains uncertain.

Thromboprophylaxis in Elective Spine Surgery for Degenerative Disease/Deformity

Patients with No Prophylaxis

Earlier studies in which venography was used as the primary follow-up method reported a postoperative DVT incidence of up to 18 % in patients who were not receiving thromboprophylaxis. In a study performed in 1994, the highest DVT rate, 27 %, was obtained in a group of patients undergoing elective lumbar spine surgery under spinal anesthesia (14 %, general anesthesia). In comparison, more recent studies have described lower DVT rates in patients who had no prophylaxis and a diagnosis of DVT based on clinical examination (1.6 %) [6, 7]. As was reported in a recent systematic review, the overall incidence is approximately 2.7 % [7, 30]. According to the authors, some of the factors that can lead to poorer results are a larger number of fused vertebral levels, greater estimated blood loss, side of the surgical approach (ipsilateral limb affected), and duration of convalescence in bed. Most of the studies included retrospective cohorts. Few of them described the true incidence of PE (very low), the data seemed to be biased, and the correlation with DVT was not specified. Oda et al. carried out a prospective clinical trial in 134 patients undergoing spine surgery, in whom prophylaxis was not performed, but postoperative venography screening was done [31]. None of the patients showed clinical signs of VTE, but radiographic signs were seen in 15.5 %, particularly in those with lumbar surgery (statistically significant difference with respect to cervical surgery). Differences were also found in relation to the patient's age. The authors concluded that the prevalence of DVT following posterior spine surgery is higher than has been generally recognized [30, 31].

Use of Mechanical Devices as the Primary Prophylaxis Method

In a series of studies carried out in the 1990s by the same research team using color Doppler follow-up and elastic compression stockings as the primary prophylaxis method, the reported DVT rate was 5–6 %. The overall conclusion of this effort was that intermittent pneumatic compression use significantly lowered the DVT rate, but there were no differences in relation to the duration of surgery, type of intervention, days immobilized, or smoking habit.

In studies applying IPC, the documented incidence of DVT ranges from 3 to 6 % [30]. However, these research efforts were performed in patients with various conditions, the incidence of PE was not always clearly stated, and the methods used to diagnose DVT differed between studies. Device use versus no prophylaxis and general versus spinal anesthesia seemed to significantly decrease the risk of DVT (6 % as a general rate) in a prospective study of 211 elective lumbar surgery patients, in whom venography was used as the diagnostic test [30].

In the review of eight studies (one randomized prospective, two comparative prospective, three prospective cohorts, and two retrospective cohorts), IPC plus thigh-length compression stockings were used as primary prophylaxis following various types of spine surgery (major reconstruction, lumbar laminectomy, tumors, degenerative disease). Doppler ultrasound was the diagnostic screening method, and the incidence of DVT was 0.0–9.8 %, and PE 0.0–1 %. In one study involving additional use of perfusion ventilation CT for the diagnosis, the incidence of PE was 2.6 % [6, 30].

Based on these findings, the incidence of DVT seems to be lower in patients treated with IPC and elastic compression stockings in comparison to other prophylaxis methods, but in the studies reporting this conclusion, DVTs were mainly detected at the distal level of the knee, and the clinical significance of this finding is uncertain.

Pharmacologic Anticoagulants

The risk of bleeding related to anticoagulant use in spine surgery was low in a review [6] of five prospective studies and one retrospective cohort. Focusing on major bleeding, the rate was 0–4.3 % [6]. One of the studies included in the review comparatively evaluated 110 patients undergoing major surgery of the spine divided into three groups, one receiving standard compression stockings, another with added pneumatic compression, and a third in which warfarin treatment was additionally given perioperatively to maintain prothrombin time at 1.3–1.5 times the control value. Bleeding complications were only seen in the warfarin-treated patients: increased bleeding through the drains on the first postoperative day in one patient (minor bleeding) and increased intraoperative bleeding in another (major bleeding). Doppler ultrasound was the diagnostic method used for follow-up, and no other adverse effects were documented. Another prospective study was undertaken in 179 patients with lumbar disc prolapse, randomized into two groups, one receiving 32 mg of LMWH/day and placebo and the other receiving 5,000 IU of UFH twice daily. All patients were given 0.5 mg of dihydroergotamine. Medication was given 2 h before surgery and every 12 h postoperatively for at least 1 week. The incidence of major intraoperative bleeding was 4.3 % in the LMWH group, compared to no cases in patients treated with UFH. Increased postoperative bleeding was reported in 9.2 % of patients receiving LMWH and 3.3 % of those with UFH and a higher percentage of patients treated with LMWH required transfusion (5.7 vs. 4.3 %). There were no differences between the groups in the percentages of hematomas, other adverse effects, or deaths. In a comparable study with regard to the disease examined and method used, but with a smaller sample (50 patients), UFH 2,500 IU was given every 12 h versus placebo. Intraoperative bleeding was lower in the placebo group (28 %) than in patients treated with heparin (24 %). There was one case of spinal hematoma in the placebo group that resolved spontaneously.

Bemiparin administration was reviewed in a prospective multicenter cohort of 231 patients undergoing spine surgery, who received 3,500 or 2,500 IU subcutaneously/day for a mean of 3 weeks. Major bleeding complications (bleeding in a vital organ, bleeding requiring surgery, massive hemorrhage, or bleeding requiring treatment discontinuation) occurred in 0.89 % of patients, and 3.56 % experienced an episode of minor bleeding. Another prospective cohort of 270 consecutive patients undergoing spine surgery analyzed the use of compression stockings plus 20 mg/day of enoxaparin starting 8 h after completion of the procedure and continuing up to the third postoperative day, with administration of 40 mg/day thereafter. Postoperative hematoma requiring urgent spinal decompression developed on two occasions (0.7 %). None of the patients presented neurological signs or symptoms.

In the case of nadroparin calcium, perioperative antithrombotic prophylaxis with compression stockings plus prompt administration of 0.3 mL (2,850 IU) of this anticoagulant drug (within 24 h postoperatively) was analyzed in a retrospective cohort of 1,954 consecutive patients. Major postoperative bleeding, defined as surgical wound hematoma causing refractory pain or epidural hematoma with a spinal mass effect diagnosed by magnetic resonance imaging (MRI), occurred in 0.7 and 0.4 % of surgical procedures, respectively, following nadroparin administration. The hematomas were immediately evacuated, and 0.2 % of patients had a residual neurological deficit [6].

Agnelli et al. performed a randomized, double-blind, multicenter clinical trial to determine the risk of VTE in patients undergoing cranial or spinal surgery [32]. Among the total, 139 patients had prophylactic graduated compression stockings, and 130 had stockings plus enoxaparin 40 mg/day starting 24 h after the intervention. Only one patient belonging to the group without LMWH had an episode of PE. Nonetheless, diagnostic screening with venography disclosed a statistically significant incidence of DVT (30 and 22 %, respectively in both groups), demonstrating a risk reduction in patients treated with anticoagulants. Considering that the risk-benefit of anticoagulant treatment in both procedures is similar with respect to morbidity and probability of bleeding complications, conclusions for the spine surgery group can be extrapolated from the overall results, although the data were not reported separately [32].

Postoperative Epidural Hematoma

The possibility of developing postoperative epidural hematoma (PEH) with prophylactic heparin use should be weighed against the benefits of preventing a thromboembolic event. It is difficult to establish the risk of PEH following spine surgery or the influence of heparin use on the development of this condition. We do not have precise knowledge of the incidence of symptomatic PEH owing to the uncertainty regarding the real versus the perceived risk of developing this complication. A systematic review of articles reporting the incidence of symptomatic PEH showed a range of 0–0.7 % in studies in which patients received pharmacological prophylaxis and 0–1 % in the overall studies. The incidence of clinically relevant epidural hematoma did not exceed 1 % in any study [33].

The catastrophic morbidity related to symptomatic PEH is a strong deterrent to initiation of pharmacological prophylaxis after spine surgery, and the available published data do not suffice to establish its safety. Most authors affirm that the use of therapeutic heparin doses postoperatively in spine surgery patients who present PE is associated with a higher incidence of bleeding complications.

A critical question is whether the use of anticoagulant thromboprophylaxis will increase the risk of symptomatic epidural hematoma. Three fundamentals should be established in this question: define patients at a high risk of VTE, determine the priority of anticoagulant treatment in patients who have received anticoagulants previously for their underlying disease, and establish the safe period for starting anticoagulant therapy when a postoperative event occurs, such as DVT, PE, acute myocardial infarction, or a nonhemorrhagic cerebrovascular accident. With respect to the first issue, if the incidence of epidural hematoma in patients treated with LMWH following spine surgery does not exceed 0.7 %, as is reported in the literature, it would seem correct to affirm that pharmacological prophylaxis is a safe choice but with caution and not as the standard of care. Given the dearth of randomized studies on this topic, the application of conclusions to the general population is very limited. As to the other two issues, the limited available data proceed from case series, and clear recommendations cannot be established.

Considering asymptomatic PEH, an incidence of up to 58 % in patients undergoing lumbar decompression has been reported when MRI examination is used within 2–5 days following the procedure. Furthermore, up to 89 % of asymptomatic epidural hematomas with no clinical repercussions have been cited in patients without drains and 36 % in those with drains, diagnosed by MRI [34].

Vertebral Trauma

The hypercoagulability state induced by traumatic injury, together with other factors such as obesity and prolonged immobilization, increases the VTE risk in patients with vertebral fracture/luxation [15]. The reported incidences of thromboembolic events in this population differ considerably, depending on the study methods. In a retrospective study by Dai et al. in 143 patients with thoracolumbar burst fracture, the incidence of VTE was 2.1 %, and there were no significant differences between those treated surgically or not [5]. The prophylaxis options in patients with spine trauma have been investigated in only one prospective study: Kurtoglu et al. analyzed 120 patients with severe head trauma and spinal injury, randomized into two groups, one with mechanical prophylaxis (IPC) and the other with IPC plus 40 mg of enoxaparin/day, starting 24 h following hospital admission. The overall incidence of DVT was 5.8 % and PE 5 % (particularly affecting patients with known DVT), with no significant differences between the two groups. There was no increase in cranial epidural hematoma on CT and no spinal epidural hematoma on subjective assessment [5].

Thromboprophylaxis in Patients with an Acute Spinal Cord Lesion

Patients with SCI who do not receive prophylaxis have the highest incidence of DVT of all hospitalized patients. Asymptomatic DVT is documented in 60–100 % of those who undergo routine screening, and PE is the third cause of death in this population [7]. The factors associated with a higher incidence of DVT are advanced age, paraplegia versus tetraplegia, severity of the lesion (complete versus incomplete), concomitant lower limb fractures, neoplastic disease, and delay in the start of thromboprophylaxis. Venous thrombosis following SCI results in considerable dysfunction at long term. These patients have a low incidence of venous recanalization after DVT, and they are candidates for major bleeding complications associated with prolonged anticoagulation. A small number of randomized clinical trials have suggested that UFH or IPC used alone is insufficient in a patient with SCI, whereas LMWH would be considerably more effective. A randomized controlled study including 476 patients compared two prophylaxis methods: one group received UFH 5,000 IU/8 h plus IPC, and the other LMWH (enoxaparin) 30 mg every 12 h. The incidence of DVT diagnosed by venography was 62 and 63 %, respectively, whereas major complications (proximal DVT and PE) developed in 16 and 12 % of patients. Major bleeding complications were observed in 5 and 3 % of patients in the two groups, respectively, without significant differences [35]. Although the period of greatest thromboembolic risk after SCI is the acute phase, DVT, PE, or fatal PE can also occur in the rehabilitation phase, even with the use of heparin. DVT rates of 8–22 % (more common with UFH) have been described in this phase.

The high thromboembolic risk in SCI patients and the existing evidence advocate prompt use of pharmacological prophylaxis in all cases. UFH or mechanical prophylaxis methods alone would not suffice. The most highly indicated would be LMWH or LMWH (preferable) versus UFH plus an IPC mechanism, started promptly. Following hospital admission, the patient should undergo a primary hemostasis study, and when normal status is confirmed, anticoagulant treatment can be started. In the case of a bleeding disorder, mechanical prophylaxis alone is started until the risk of bleeding decreases, and pharmacological prophylaxis can be added. For late DVT prevention, LMWH or AVK therapy should be continued during rehabilitation for minimum of 3 months. In patients with incomplete SCI and a spinal hematoma diagnosed by CT or MRI, initiation of LMWH treatment should be postponed for 1–3 days. If total anticoagulation with coumarins is needed, the treatment should be delayed for at least 1 week because of the unpredictable response to dosing with these agents [34].

Even in patients with a high thromboembolic risk, such as those with cord lesions, a recent study reviewing asymptomatic DVT in SCI patients failed to find sufficient evidence to support or negate routine screening for DVT in adults with traumatic SCI receiving anticoagulant treatment [36].

Conclusions

Thromboprophylaxis in trauma patients is considered a quality standard in health care. Resources should be devoted to developing and implementing robust protocols in this setting. In most trauma patients, thromboprophylaxis with LMWH can be started at 48 h, and in patients with active bleeding, mechanical compression should be considered, despite its limited effectiveness, until the risk of hemorrhage has decreased. Generally speaking, thromboprophylaxis with LMWH is more effective than IPC.

In elective spinal surgery (degenerative, deformity, infection), the thromboembolic risk is relatively low, and the use of mechanical devices as primary prophylaxis seems reasonable. The currently available evidence does not suffice to support or negate the use of anticoagulant agents in this surgery, but it does exclude routine application, based on the low risk of fatal pulmonary embolism. These agents are, however, appropriate for patients with significant neurological dysfunction (e.g., SCI patients) who require lengthy bed rest. When heparin is used, the wound and the patient's neurological function should be carefully monitored. Again, there is not enough data to justify routine screening with ultrasound or venography in patients who have undergone this surgery.

Multimodal treatment (mechanical and pharmacological) that guarantees optimal thromboprophylaxis in this type of patient currently implies a rational, multidisciplinary decision, supported by evidence-based medicine.

Key points – recommendations

Multiple trauma	Head trauma
When LMWH is contraindicated because of active bleeding or a high bleeding risk, mechanical methods are recommended (IPC or compression stockings alone, grade 1B)	The Brain Trauma Foundation recommendations include the use of mechanical prophylaxis with GCS or IPC in all head trauma patients until they are ambulatory, unless there is lower limb injury and this measure cannot be applied
When the risk of bleeding decreases, reintroduction of thromboprophylaxis is recommended (grade 1C)	It is recommended to prolong thromboprophylaxis until hospital discharge (grade 1C), and if mobility is decreased, to continue prophylaxis (grade 2C)
LMWH administration can be combined with mechanical methods (grade 1B)	Initiation of thromboprophylaxis is delayed until there is no risk of hemorrhage with active bleeding (subdural/epidural/intracerebral hematoma); minimum 48 h
In patients with a high risk of VTE with or without suboptimal prophylaxis (grade 1C), Doppler ultrasound screening is recommended	In patients with a high risk of VTE with or without suboptimal thromboprophylaxis (grade 1C), Doppler ultrasound screening is recommended
IVC filters are not recommended for prophylaxis (grade 1C)	IVC filters are not recommended for prophylaxis (grade 1C)

Refs. [7, 26]

LMWH low molecular weight heparin, *IPC* intermittent pneumatic compression, *VTE* venous thromboembolic disease, *IVC* inferior vena cava, *GCS* graduated compression stockings

Key points – recommendations

Elective spine surgery	Acute cord lesion
In patients with no thromboembolic risk factors, routine thromboprophylaxis use is not recommended with the exception of prompt, frequent ambulation (grade 2C)	Routine thromboprophylaxis is recommended in all patients with SCI (grade 1A). LMWH should be started after evaluating the patient's primary hemostasis (grade 1B). An alternative would be combined use of IPC and UFH (grade 1B) or LMWH (grade 1C)
In patients with risk factors, such as advanced age, neoplastic disease, neurological deficit, previous DVT, or an anterior surgical approach, low-dose postoperative UFH (grade 1B), LMWH (Grade 1B), or optimal perioperative IPC use (grade 1B) are recommended. As an alternative option, GCS (grade 2B)	For SCI patients, optimal IPC and/or GCS use is recommended when anticoagulant thromboprophylaxis is contraindicated due to a high risk of bleeding following the injury (grade 1A). When the risk decreases, pharmacologic thromboprophylaxis can be added or replace the mechanical method (grade 1C)
In patients with multiple risk factors, a pharmacological method is suggested (UFH or LMWH) combined with optimal use of a mechanical method (GCS and/or IPC) (grade 2C)	In patients with incomplete SCI associated with radiologic evidence (CT or MRI) of spinal hematoma, mechanical thromboprophylaxis is recommended instead of prophylactic anticoagulants at least in the first days following the injury (grade 1C)
It is suggested that use of compression devices on the lower limbs in elective spine procedures should be initiated just before the start of surgery and continued until the patient is completely ambulatory. Pharmacological prophylaxis is not justified in most elective spine surgeries performed thorough a posterior approach	In patients undergoing rehabilitation after SCI, continuation of thromboprophylaxis with LMWH or conversion to oral AVK is recommended (target INR 2.5, range 2.0–3.0) (grade 1C)
LMWH or UFH can be used after combined elective posterior-anterior spine surgery or in patients identified as having a high risk of thromboembolism (e.g., multiple trauma, malignancy, or hypercoagulability states) (NASS recommendations)	IVC filters are excluded for thromboprophylaxis in patients with SCI (grade 1C)
	Exclusive use of UFH following SCI is excluded (grade 1A)

Refs. [7, 34]

DVT deep venous thrombosis, *UFH* nonfractionated heparin, *LMWH* low molecular weight heparin, *IPC* intermittent pneumatic compression, *GCS* graduated compression stockings, *NASS* North American Spine Society, *SCI* acute spinal cord injury, *CT* computed tomography, *MRI* magnetic resonance imaging, *AVK* antivitamin K, *IVC* inferior vena cava

References

1. Velmahos GC. The current status of thromboprophylaxis after trauma: a story of confusion and uncertainty. Am Surg. 2006;72:757–63.
2. Velmahos GC. Posttraumatic thromboprophylaxis revisited: an argument against the current methods of DVT and PE prophylaxis after injury. World J Surg. 2006;30:483–7.

3. Ploumis A, Ponnappan RK, Sarbello J, Dvorak M, Fehlings MG, Baron E, et al. Thromboprophylaxis in traumatic and elective spinal surgery: analysis of questionnaire response and current practice of spine trauma surgeons. Spine (Phila Pa 1976). 2010; 35:323–9.

4. Ploumis A, Ponnappan RK, Bessey JT, Patel R, Vaccaro AR. Thromboprophylaxis in spinal trauma surgery: consensus among spine trauma surgeons. Spine J. 2009;9:530–6.

5. Heck CA, Brown CR, Richardson WJ. Venous thromboembolism in spine surgery. J Am Acad Orthop Surg. 2008;16:656–64.

6. Cheng JS, Arnold PM, Anderson PA, Fischer D, Dettori JR. Anticoagulation risk in spine surgery. Spine (Phila Pa 1976). 2010;35:S117–24.

7. Geerts WH, Bergqvist D, Pineo GF, Heit JA, Samama CM, Lassen MR, et al. Prevention of venous thromboembolism: American College of Chest Physicians evidence-based clinical practice guidelines (8th edition). Chest. 2008;133:381S–453.

8. Latronico N, Berardino M. Thromboembolic prophylaxis in head trauma and multiple-trauma patients. Minerva Anestesiol. 2008;74:543–8.

9. Knudson MM, Ikossi DG, Khaw L, Morabito D, Speetzen LS. Thromboembolism after trauma: an analysis of 1602 episodes from the American College of Surgeons National Trauma Data Bank. Ann Surg. 2004;240:490–6.

10. Van Stralen KJ, Rosendaal FR, Doggen CJ. Minor injuries as a risk factor for venous thrombosis. Arch Intern Med. 2008;168:21–6.

11. Dudley RR, Aziz I, Bonnici A, Saluja RS, Lamoureux J, Kalmovitch B, et al. Early venous thromboembolic event prophylaxis in traumatic brain injury with low-molecular-weight heparin: risks and benefits. J Neurotrauma. 2010;27:2165–72.

12. Page RB, Spott MA, Krishnamurthy S, Taleghani C, Chinchilli VM. Head injury and pulmonary embolism: a retrospective report based on the Pennsylvania Trauma Outcomes study. Neurosurgery. 2004;54:143–8.

13. Yenna ZC, Roberts C. Thromboprophylaxis after multiple trauma: what treatment and for how long? Injury. 2009;40 Suppl 4:S90–4.

14. Paffrath T, Wafaisade A, Lefering R, Simanski C, Bouillon B, Spanholtz T, et al. Venous thromboembolism after severe trauma: incidence, risk factors and outcome. Injury. 2010; 41:97–101.

15. Meissner MH, Chandler WL, Elliott JS. Venous thromboembolism in trauma: a local manifestation of systemic hypercoagulability? J Trauma. 2003;54:224–31.

16. Rogers FB, Cipolle MD, Velmahos G, Rozycki G, Luchette FA. Practice management guidelines for the prevention of venous thromboembolism in trauma patients: the EAST practice management guidelines work group. J Trauma. 2002;53:142–64.

17. Shakur H, Roberts I, Bautista R, Caballero J, Coats T, Dewan Y, et al. Effects of tranexamic acid on death, vascular occlusive events, and blood transfusion in trauma patients with significant haemorrhage (CRASH-2): a randomised, placebo-controlled trial. Lancet. 2010;376:23–32.

18. Knudson MM, Ikossi DG. Venous thromboembolism after trauma. Curr Opin Crit Care. 2004;10:539–48.

19. Gersin K, Grindlinger GA, Lee V, Dennis RC, Wedel SK, Cachecho R. The efficacy of sequential compression devices in multiple trauma patients with severe head injury. J Trauma. 1994;37:205–8.

20. Davidson JE, Willms DC, Hoffman MS. Effect of intermittent pneumatic leg compression on intracranial pressure in brain-injured patients. Crit Care Med. 1993;21:224–7.

21. Ginzburg E, Cohn SM, Lopez J, Jackowski J, Brown M, Hameed SM. Randomized clinical trial of intermittent pneumatic compression and low molecular weight heparin in trauma. Br J Surg. 2003;90:1338–44.

22. Lacut K, Bressollette L, Le GG, Etienne E, De TA, Renault A, et al. Prevention of venous thrombosis in patients with acute intracerebral hemorrhage. Neurology. 2005;65:865–9.

23. Alejandro KV, Acosta JA, Rodriguez PA. Bleeding manifestations after early use of low-molecular-weight heparins in blunt splenic injuries. Am Surg. 2003;69:1006–9.

24. Koehler DM, Shipman J, Davidson MA, Guillamondegui O. Is early venous thromboembolism prophylaxis safe in trauma patients with intracranial hemorrhage. J Trauma. 2011;70: 324–9.
25. Reiff DA, Haricharan RN, Bullington NM, Griffin RL, McGwin Jr G, Rue III LW. Traumatic brain injury is associated with the development of deep vein thrombosis independent of pharmacological prophylaxis. J Trauma. 2009;66:1436–40.
26. Brain Trauma Foundation; American Association of Neurological Surgeons; Congress of Neurological Surgeons. Guidelines for the management of severe traumatic brain injury. J Neurotrauma. 2007;24 Suppl 1:S1–106.
27. Bratton SL, Chestnut RM, Ghajar J, McConnell Hammond FF, Harris OA, Hartl R, et al. Guidelines for the management of severe traumatic brain injury. V. deep vein thrombosis prophylaxis. J Neurotrauma. 2007;24 Suppl 1:S32–6.
28. Norwood SH, Berne JD, Rowe SA, Villarreal DH, Ledlie JT. Early venous thromboembolism prophylaxis with enoxaparin in patients with blunt traumatic brain injury. J Trauma. 2008;65:1021–6.
29. Rosner MK, Kuklo TR, Tawk R, Moquin R, Ondra SL. Prophylactic placement of an inferior vena cava filter in high-risk patients undergoing spinal reconstruction. Neurosurg Focus. 2004;17:E6.
30. Glotzbecker MP, Bono CM, Wood KB, Harris MB. Thromboembolic disease in spinal surgery: a systematic review. Spine (Phila Pa 1976). 2009;34:291–303.
31. Oda T, Fuji T, Kato Y, Fujita S, Kanemitsu N. Deep venous thrombosis after posterior spinal surgery. Spine (Phila Pa 1976). 2000;25:2962–7.
32. Agnelli G, Piovella F, Buoncristiani P, Severi P, Pini M, D'Angelo A, et al. Enoxaparin plus compression stockings compared with compression stockings alone in the prevention of venous thromboembolism after elective neurosurgery. N Engl J Med. 1998;339:80–5.
33. Glotzbecker MP, Bono CM, Wood KB, Harris MB. Postoperative spinal epidural hematoma: a systematic review. Spine (Phila Pa 1976). 2010;35:E413–20.
34. Bono CM, Watters WC, Heggeness MH, Resnick DK, Shaffer WO, Baiden J et al. Antithrombotic therapies in spine surgery. In: North American Spine Society, editor. North American Spine Society evidence-based clinical guidelines for multidisciplinary spine care. Burr Ridge: North American Spine Society; 2009. p. 17–21.
35. Spinal Cord Injury Thromboprophylaxis Investigators. Prevention of venous thromboembolism in the acute treatment phase after spinal cord injury: a randomized, multicenter trial comparing low-dose heparin plus intermittent pneumatic compression with enoxaparin. J Trauma. 2003;54:1116–24.
36. Furlan JC, Fehlings MG. Role of screening tests for deep venous thrombosis in asymptomatic adults with acute spinal cord injury: an evidence-based analysis. Spine (Phila Pa 1976). 2007;32:1908–16.

Chapter 12
Management of Antiaggregated and Anticoagulated Patients Scheduled for Orthopedic Surgery

Raquel Ferrandis and Juan V. Llau

Abstract Patients undergoing surgery are more and more frequent under the effects of antiplatelet agents or anticoagulant drugs. This situation is a challenge for the surgical team, and their management is of capital importance to avoid bleeding (the risk of bleeding is increased if the hemostasis is not maintained) and thrombosis (the risk to develop venous or arterial thrombi is increased when the anticlotting drugs are stopped).

Recently, many new drugs have been introduced to raise the efficacy of therapies against the thrombotic development, difficulting the optimal management of patients in the perioperative period. In this chapter, we give an actual overview of this scenario introducing the most recent recommendations for this situation, specifically addressed for patients scheduled for orthopedic surgery.

Keywords Anticoagulants • Antiplatelets • Hemorrhagic risk • Thrombotic risk Perioperative management

R. Ferrandis, M.D., Ph.D. (✉)
Department of Anesthesiology and Critical Care,
Hospital Clinic Universitari de València,
Avda Blasco Ibáñez 17,
46006 Valencia, Spain

Department of Human Physiology, School of Medicine, Valencia University,
Valencia, Spain
e-mail: raquelferrandis@gmail.com

J.V. Llau
Department of Anesthesiology and Critical Care,
Hospital Clinic Universitari de València,
Avda Blasco Ibáñez 17, 46006 Valencia, Spain

Human Physiology and Anesthesiology,
School of Medicine, Catholic Uniersity "San Vicente Martir",
Valencia, Spain
e-mail: juanvllau@gmail.com

J.V. Llau (ed.), *Thromboembolism in Orthopedic Surgery*,
DOI 10.1007/978-1-4471-4336-9_12, © Springer-Verlag London 2013

Introduction

Orthopedic surgery is performed in many cases in patients which are under the effect of some drugs. Most common drugs are, probably, antiplatelet and anticoagulant agents. The management of these patients is a common challenging problem and a cause of frequent assessment from orthopedic surgeons. These patients could require temporary interruption of the administration of the antiplatelet or anticoagulant drug, being necessary to balance the risk of a thromboembolic event during the interruption of the therapy with the risk for bleeding when the antithrombotic drug is administered too close to surgery.

Current guidelines for the management of these patients are revised, but because one of the most important challenges is the patient with fracture of the neck of the femur, we will review also these specific patients.

Antiplatelet Agents

It is very common that patients who are scheduled for orthopedic surgery are treated with antiplatelet agents (APA) due to their wide indications and the characteristics of these patients. They are several possibilities of treatment, and patients can be under the effect of acetylsalicylic acid (ASA) alone, one thienopyridine alone (the most common is clopidogrel, but we are going to find patients in a near future with other thienopyridines, as prasugrel or ticagrelor), or, in selected cases, the combination of them.

Main challenges for the anesthesiologist and the orthopedic surgeon include patients with a coronary stent (mainly, drug-eluting coronary stents), urgent surgery, and patients with fracture of the neck of the femur. We will review current protocols and discuss most recent proposals for the management of APA in these patients.

The APA are drugs of diverse origin, whose prophylactic and therapeutic effects are especially important in the prevention and treatment of the arterial thrombosis. The current indications of APA include cardiac and neurologic diseases; one brief summary of the most important of them is shown in Table 12.1 [1–7].

All APA are able to inhibit platelet function, particularly activation and subsequent aggregation, although they produce this effect through different ways showing different antiplatelet activity (Table 12.2) [8, 9]. APA can be classified into four groups, depending on their mechanisms of action.

Antiplatelet agents which antagonize the adenosine diphosphate (ADP) receptor, such as the thienopyridine compounds ticlopidine and clopidogrel. They reach their peak of activity after 3–5 days and produce a prolonged antiplatelet effect (7–10 days) due to its long half-life. New ADP receptor antagonists include prasugrel (a thienopyridine) and ticagrelor. As with clopidogrel, prasugrel is a prodrug that requires hepatic conversion and a loading dose to shorten the onset of platelet inhibition. Ticagrelor produces a reversible action with a peak of antiaggregation at 2–3 h after its oral administration.

Table 12.1 Some recognized indications for the administration of the antiplatelet drugs

Indications in cardiology	Acute coronary syndrome
	Stable angina
	Unstable angina/acute myocardial infarction without Q wave
	Percutaneous coronary angioplasty (with/without coronary stent placement)
	Patients after coronary bypass surgery
	Selected patients with atrial fibrillation and/or valvulopathies
Indications in neurology	Acute phase of the stroke
	Secondary prevention of the stroke
Other potential indications	Patient of valve prosthesis
	Emboligen carotid stenosis
	Carotid endarterectomy
	Patients with antiphospholipid antibodies
	Peripheral arteriopathy with or without intermittent claudication
	Primary prevention in patients with cardiovascular risk

Table 12.2 Antiaggregant effect of some of the antiplatelet agents

Mechanism of action	Antiplatelet agent	Length of action	Recommended time of discontinuation until reaching hemostatic competence
Inhibition of cyclooxygenase 1 enzyme	Aspirin	7 days	3 days (2–5 days)
	Several NSAIDs	Variable (1–7 days)	Variable
Antagonism of ADP receptor	Ticlopidine	10 days	7 days
	Clopidogrel	7 days	5 days (3–7 days)
	Ticagrelor	5 days	3 days (2–5 days)
	Prasugrel	10 days	7 days
Increase of intraplatelet levels of cAPM	Dipyridamole	24 h	24 h

Agents which antagonize the GPIIb/IIIa receptors, of exclusively intravenous use, which are more powerful, albeit with a shorter-lasting action (24 h) are eptifibatide, abciximab, and tirofiban.

Agents which increase the intraplatelet levels of AMPc are as follows: The best known agent is dipyridamole (moderate antiplatelet effect lasting about 24 h). Other agents are the I-2 prostaglandin (epoprostenol) and its analog iloprost, both used intravenously with a brief antiplatelet effect (<3 h).

Inhibitors of cyclooxygenase 1 enzyme (COX-1) are as follows: The best known are acetylsalicylic acid (ASA) and non-steroidal anti-inflammatory drugs (NSAIDs). ASA is the most deeply studied and its antiplatelet effect takes place with the irreversible blockade of COX-1, so its action lasts through-out all the life of the platelet (7–10 days). Nevertheless, there is enough number of platelets to guarantee suitable hemostasis from the third to fourth day. The NSAIDs also produce inhibition of platelet aggregation by a similar mecha-nism to the ASA, although there are two important aspects to bear in mind: Firstly, the blocking effect of the COX-1 is reversible, thus once the drug has been eliminated, the platelet function is restored and, secondly, the different capacity of all the NSAIDs to inhibit COX-1 and, consequently, in their anti-platelet action.

General Considerations on the Treatment of APA [7–13]

The role of aspirin in the primary prevention has extended its prescription based on related factors of cardiovascular and/or neurological risk. Moreover, the combina-tion of two APA (mainly ASA and clopidogrel) in high-risk patients is a more and more extended practice.

Dual antiplatelet therapy must be maintained at least 12 months after drug-eluting stent placement, and elective surgery must be postponed. If surgery cannot be postponed, at least ASA should be continued if at all possible through-out the perioperative period so that the patient is operated under its antiplatelet effect and the thienopyridine should be restarted as soon as possible after that procedure.

The interindividual response to the APA is evident, and it can be modified by several factors such as patient's compliance, dose, smoking, exercise, concomitant medications, heart failure, hyperlipidemia, or hyperglucemia, and a valid universal pattern of antiplatelet management for all patients seems not to exist.

In most orthopedic surgery, the current attitude is to maintain APA therapy throughout the perioperative period if the patient has a moderate to high thrombotic risk. The main reason for this recommendation is that APA cessation has proved to be an independent factor *per se* of death and major cardiac events.

Main Recommendations for Patients Scheduled for Orthopedic Surgery

The practical guidelines for the management of APA on patients scheduled for elec-tive orthopedic surgery need the local agreement between anesthesiologists and orthopedic surgeons, with the participation and acceptance by hematologists, cardi-ologists, and neurologists.

Our proposal is to classify the orthopedic procedures in three steps:

- *Major Hemorrhage Risk*. Orthopedic procedures with bleeding risk in an enclosed space: spinal surgery

- *Moderate Hemorrhage Risk*. Orthopedic procedures in which transfusion is usually needed: total knee or hip arthroplasty, fracture of the neck of the femur, and some procedures in trauma patients
- *Minor Hemorrhagic Risk*. Orthopedic procedures in which the need for transfusion is unlikely: arthroscopy, minor procedures, biopsies, etc.

The following general recommendations can be suggested [8–16]:

- *Elective Surgery of High Hemorrhagic Risk*

  - Elective high-risk hemorrhagic surgery has to be delayed if thrombotic risk is high: recent (less than 6 weeks) myocardial infarction, cardiac surgery, placement of a bare metal stent, cerebrovascular stroke, or less than 12 months after the placement of a drug-eluting coronary stent.
  - In patients with moderate thrombotic risk (between 6 and 36 weeks in the first group of pathologies and 12–18 months after the placement of a drug-eluting stent), and the performance of high hemorrhagic risk surgery is mandatory, the main recommendation is to maintain ASA until 2–3 days before surgery and to give it after surgery as soon as possible.
  - If the neurologic and cardiovascular risk is low or the prescription of the APA is for "primary prevention," the APA should be withdrawn (7 days for ASA, 10 days for clopidogrel).

- *Elective Surgery of Moderate Hemorrhagic Risk*

  - If thrombotic risk is high, surgery should be postponed, but if not, the maintenance of ASA is mandatory, and clopidogrel can be maintained or stopped 3–5 days prior to surgery.
  - When the thrombotic risk is intermediate, the agreement is similar: maintenance of ASA until the day before surgery (if the APA is another one, it has to be substituted by ASA around 10 days before) and administration of the first dose after surgery not more than 24 h once surgery has finished.

- *Elective Surgery of Low Hemorrhagic Risk*

  - Although it is also recommended to delay surgery if thrombotic risk is high, in general, ASA can be maintained until surgery.
  - If the patient is under treatment with a thienopyridine, we can replace it by ASA and maintain it.
  - If a dual therapy is necessary, the recommendation is to maintain ASA and to stop clopidogrel 5 days before surgery.

- *Surgery of the Fracture of the Neck of the Femur*

  - The main recommendation is not to wait 7–10 days to perform the surgery if the patient is under the effect of ASA or under the effect of clopidogrel.
  - Surgery should be performed when the patient is stable (hemodynamic and medical compensation of its comorbidities should be reached before surgery).
  - The most common recommendation is to perform surgery 2–3 days after the fracture although the patient has taken any APA, but this suggestion should be accorded by the surgical team.

Anticoagulant Drugs

The perioperative management of patients scheduled for orthopedic surgery that are receiving vitamin K antagonists (VKAs) and require temporary interruption of these drugs is a common and challenging clinical problem. Most patients receive oral and chronic anticoagulation due to atrial fibrillation or a mechanical heart valve, although other indications for it include cerebrovascular pathology (repeated strokes) or prevention of recurrences of previous thromboembolic events.

Nowadays, the anticoagulant therapy could be made by VKAs or by any of new direct oral anticoagulants (DOAC), as dabigatran, rivaroxaban or apixaban, which are recently accepted or waiting their approval for their use in this indication. The review of the management of patients scheduled for orthopedic surgery includes the VKAs and a proposal for DOAC.

Management of Patients Under the Effect Vitamin K Antagonist

The perioperative management of VKAs is well established, and nearly no change has been done in the lately recommendations [17–20]. Rational decisions are made depending on the risks of thrombosis and bleeding associated with the different alternatives. To date, there are no validated risk stratification schemes to reliably classify VKA-treated patients based on their risk for thromboembolism and bleeding. The 9th ACCP offers risk stratification schemes (Tables 12.3 and 12.4) to provide general guidance, based on indirect evidence and clinical experience [21, 22]. Nevertheless, these patients will always benefit from management according to standardized and institution-specific protocols.

In general, the interruption of VKAs is required to achieve normal or near-normal hemostasis at the time of surgery (INR 1.5 or bellow). This time must be estimated based on the elimination half-life of VKA, 8–11 h for acenocoumarol and 36–42 h for warfarin. Then, after stopping VKAs, between 3 and at least 5 days will be required for most anticoagulant effect to be eliminated. The 9th ACCP recommends in patients who require temporary interruption of a VKA before surgery, stopping VKAs approximately 5 days before surgery instead of stopping VKAs a shorter time before surgery (Grade 1C). After surgery, it is recommended resuming VKA 12–24 h postoperative, when oral intake is permitted and there is adequate hemostasis (grade 2C). In some cases with very low hemorrhagic risk, as minor dermatologic or dental procedures or cataract surgery, VKAs can be continued around the time of the procedure, optimizing the local hemostasis if necessary (recommendation grade 2C in the 9th ACCP).

The temporary discontinuation of VKAs exposes patients to a risk of thromboembolism since the INR is 1.5 before surgery till INR 2 is reached when VKAs are restarted postoperatively. Then, for patients with a mechanical heart valve, atrial fibrillation, or VTE at high risk for thromboembolism, there is a need of bridging

Table 12.3 Risk stratification for perioperative thromboembolism

Indication for VKA therapy	Risk stratum		
	High	Moderate	Low
Mechanical heart valve	Mitral valve prosthesis	Bileaflet aortic valve prosthesis + (one or more)	Bileaflet aortic valve prosthesis without atrial fibrillation and no other risk factors for stroke
	Caged-ball or tilting disc aortic valve prosthesis	Atrial fibrillation	
	Within 6 months of stroke or transient ischemic attack	Prior stroke or transient ischemic attack	
		Hypertension	
		Diabetes	
		Congestive heart failure	
		Aged over 75 years	
Atrial Fibrillation	CHADS$_2$ score 5 or 6	CHADS$_2$ score 3 or 4	CHADS$_2$ score 0–2 (assuming no prior stroke or transient ischemic attack)
	Within 3 months of stroke or transient ischemic attack		
	Rheumatic valvular heart disease		
VTE	Within 3 months of VTE	VTE within the past 3–12 months	VTE 12 months previous and no other risk factors
	Severe thrombophilia	Nonsevere thrombophilia	
		Recurrent VTE	
		Active cancer	

Table 12.4 Surgeries and procedures associated with an increased bleeding risk

Urologic surgery
  Transurethral prostate resection
  Bladder resection or tumor ablation
  Nephrectomy or kidney biopsy
Pacemaker or implantable cardioverter defibrillator device implantation
Colonic polyp resection, typically of large (i.e., 1–2 cm long) sessile polyps
Highly vascular organs, such as the kidney, liver, and spleen
Bowel resection
Major surgery with extensive tissue injury (e.g., cancer surgery, joint arthroplasty, reconstructive plastic surgery)
Cardiac, intracranial, or spinal surgery

anticoagulation (administration of a short-acting anticoagulant) during interruption of VKA therapy. On the other hand, in patients at low risk for thromboembolism, the bridging can be avoided. When there is a moderate risk for thromboembolism, the bridging or no-bridging approach chosen should be based on an assessment of

Table 12.5 Main characteristics of new oral anticoagulants

	Apixaban	Dabigatran	Rivaroxaban
Atrial fibrilation	ARISTOTLE/ AVERROES	RELY	ROCKET
	5 mg bid	110/150 mg bid	20 mg od
Treatment of thromboembolic disease (acute)	AMPLIFY 10 mg bid	RECOVER 150 mg bid	EINSTEIN 15 mg bid/20 mg od
Secondary prevention of TED	AMPLIFY EXT 2.5/5 mg bid	REMEDY 150 mg bid	EINSTEIN EXT 20 mg od
Acute coronary syndrome	APPRAISE 5 mg bid	REDEEM 50/75/110/150 mg bid	ATLAS 2.5/5 mg bid

individual patient- and surgery-related factors. If the surgery or procedures is a low risk for bleeding, the bridging may be considered; but if it is of high-bleeding risk (major cardiac surgery, carotid endarterectomy surgery), no-bridging therapy may be considered.

The bridging therapy can be performed with therapeutic-dose iv UFH or therapeutic-dose sc LMWH. Both should be stopped before surgery time enough to ensure normal hemostasis that is 4–6 h for UFH and 24 h for LMWH. After surgery, therapeutic-dose LMWH should be resumed 24 h postoperatively in non-high-bleeding-risk surgery. In patients who are undergoing high-bleeding-risk surgery, the resumption of therapeutic-dose LMWH should be delayed 48–72 h after surgery.

In nonbridging clinical settings, according to the 8th ACCP [18], clinicians may consider using low-dose LMWH for VKA-treated patients with prior VTE, in order to reduce the incidence of postoperative VTE. In these patients, low-dose LMWH will minimize the risk of postoperative major bleeding, especially for patients undergoing major surgery, with probably achieving much of the benefit of therapeutic-dose anticoagulation. However, after surgery, resumption of VKA therapy alone also may be considered as a method of prophylaxis against postoperative VTE.

New Direct Oral Anticoagulant (DOAC)

New direct oral anticoagulants, with possibilities to be used as chronic medication for anticoagulation in the current indications for warfarin or acenocumarol, are rivaroxaban, apixaban, and dabigatran. They in common are given orally, and they do not need antithrombin for their action, but they act in different targets of the coagulation cascade (Table 12.5). Several studies are being conducted with these drugs (Table 12.6), and some indications have been approved in some countries [23–28].

Table 12.6 Main dosage in studies using OAC as anticoagulant

	Apixaban	Dabigatran	Rivaroxaban
Atrial fibrillation	ARISTOTLE	RELY	ROCKET
	5 mg bid	110/150 mg bid	20 mg od
Treatment of acute	AMPLIFY	RECOVER	EINSTEIN
thromboembolic	10 mg bid	150 mg bid	15 mg bid/20 mg od
disease			
Secondary prevention	AMPLIFY EXT	REMEDY	EINSTEIN EXT
of TED	2.5/5 mg bid	150 mg bid	20 mg od
Acute coronary	APPRAISE	REDEEM	ATLAS
syndrome	5 mg bid	50–150 mg bid	2.5/5 mg bid

There is no experience about the perioperative management of new DOAC. Then, it is necessary to highlight some points before giving the recommendations:

1. There is no antidote for these drugs. Nowadays, although there are some papers with the use of PCC or factor VIIa, none of them could be considered as antidote [29, 30].
2. The dosage used for the chronic anticoagulation is quiet different to the dosage used for thromboprophylaxis. In the tables, it shows the main proposed dosage for these drugs.
3. The safety objective to be reached in patients receiving new DOAC for "full" anticoagulation is, in these days, unknown. The reason is that the use of any biological test with this objective implies the previous definition of the safety threshold; today, it is not possible to define the minimal plasmatic concentration of the drug or the range of units of anti-IIa (dabigatran) or anti-Xa (rivaroxaban or apixaban) to have the same hemorrhagic risk to a non-treated patient.

Due to the lack of experience with the management of these drugs as chronic treatment, the main objective must be the safety considered as hemorrhage associated to the surgery or the invasive procedure. Of course, the necessary antithrombotic protection should be in mind. With these initial points, the main recommendations could be divided in two:

1. Stop the Anticoagulant 4–5 Days Before Surgery and Make the Bridging with LMWH, as It Is Done with AVK
   This possibility has been proposed by the French [31] and the Spanish Anesthesiology Societies [32]. It could be the best one (the most safety one) for the three DOAC. In all cases, the treatment is stopped at least 3 times the half-life (in fact, more than three times), so the anticoagulant effect of any of them should be minimal (with 3 half-lives, the plasmatic level of the drug is less than 15 %).
   In addition, it is necessary to administrata a LMWH to bridge the anticoagulant effect (in a similar way it occurs with VKAs). The dosage of the LMWH will be based on the thrombotic risk of the patient. The last dose of LMWH will be 24 h before surgery (when anticoagulant dosage is used).

Stopping the drug 4 or 5 days before surgery are both good choices, and it could depend on the decision of each group. As general guide, the timing of stopping and administration of LMWH could be drawn as follows:

- Day 5: last intake of DOAC
- Day 4: no intake of DOAC nor LMWH
- Day 3: no intake of DOAC, administration of LMWH at the chosen dosage
- Day 2: no intake of DOAC, administration of LMWH at the chosen dosage
- Day 1 (the day before surgery): no intake of DOAC, administration of LMWH at the chosen dosage, but with the last administration 24 h before surgery
- Day 0: surgery

2. Stop the Drug Before Surgery Without Bridge

Some publications propose stopping the drug around three half-lives without the administration of LMWH. The technical specifications of rivaroxaban [33] talk of discontinuing the treatment at least 24 h. Also with dabigatran, a recently published revision proposed stopping between 1 and more than 5 days depending on the renal function and the risk of bleeding [34].

Nevertheless, this proposal could arise some doubts: It is based only on a theoretical model (the pharmacology of the drug), the time is not the same for all the drugs, and it is not possible to assure that the level of drug is as low that it will not influence on the hemorrhage in surgery. In fact, the half-life may vary depending on the renal function or the age of the patient, and it will extend the time necessary of withdrawal.

About the next dose of DOAC after surgery, if there has been a bridging with LMWH, an option would be the maintenance of LMWH during 2–3 days after surgery. Then, the beginning of the administration of the DOAC would be at third or fourth day after surgery (this day, without administration of the LMWH, the DOAC would be instead). Another option would be to start the OAC after surgery (always when the hemostasis is reached).

Hip Fracture Surgery

The management of patients with hip fracture (HF) under the effect of any anti-platelet or anticoagulant drug has the challenge to balance the benefit/risk of the delay of surgery waiting the "optimal time" related with the hemostasis against the performance of the surgery "as soon as possible" to minimize the risk related with the patient bed rest, increase of thrombotic complications, need for transfusion, etc. There is no full agreement for this situation, although most surgeons and anesthesiologists consider that the optimal time for surgery in these patients ranges between 48 and 72 h after the hip is fractured. Some possibilities could be chosen, but we propose two decision algorithms for them (Figs. 12.1 and 12.2) as the best way for their treatment. Obviously, it is only a proposal and the reader may disagree in some points, but it can be the general mark to work on.

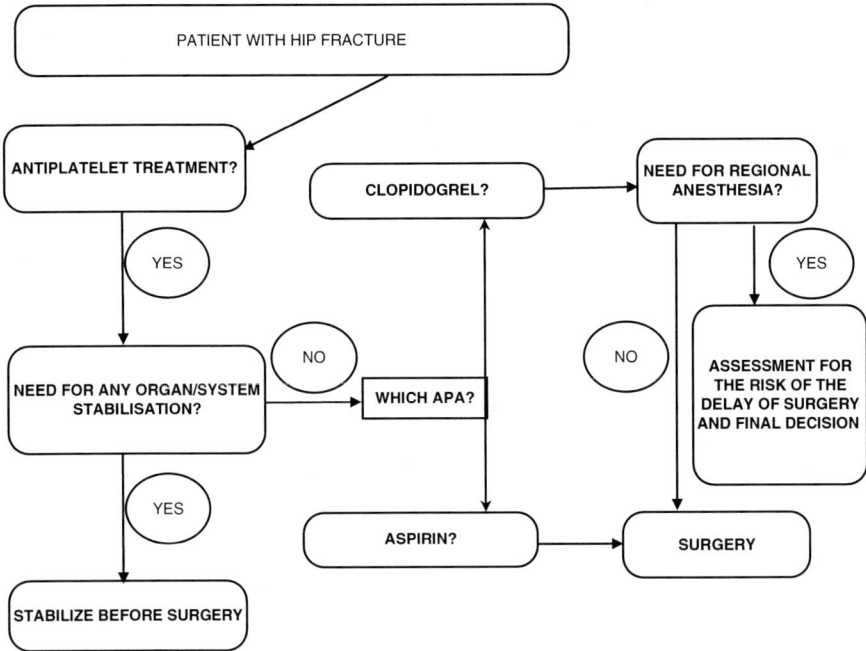

Fig. 12.1 Proposed decision algorithm for patients with hip fracture under antiplatelet (*APA*) treatment

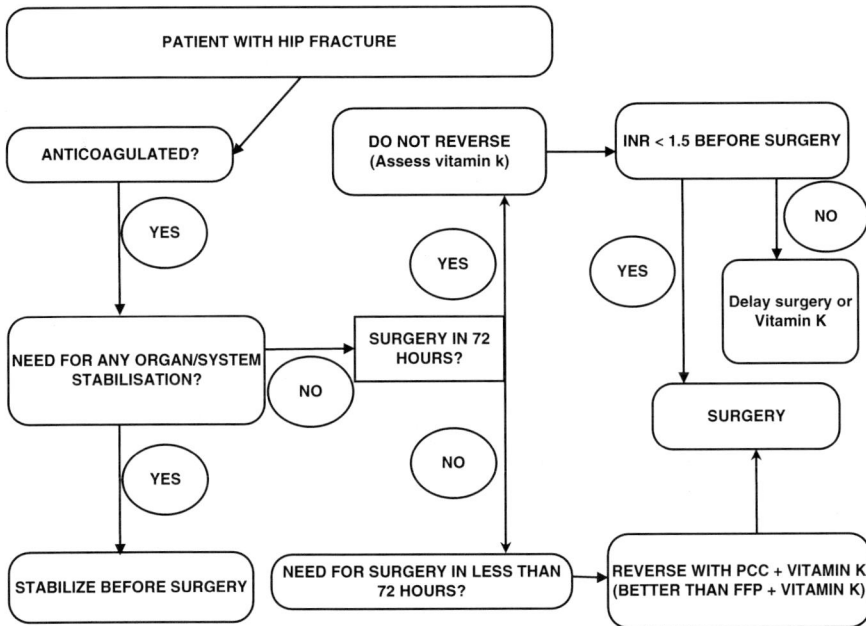

Fig. 12.2 Proposed decision algorithm for patients with hip fracture under oral anticoagulant treatment

References

1. Sobel M, Verhaeghe R. Antithrombotic therapy for peripheral artery occlusive disease: American College of Chest Physicians evidence-based clinical practice guidelines (8th edition). Chest. 2008;133(6Suppl):815S–43.
2. Becker RC, Meade TW, Berger PB, Ezekowitz M, O'Connor CM, Vorchheimer DA, et al. The primary and secondary prevention of coronary artery disease: American College of Chest Physicians evidence-based clinical practice guidelines (8th edition). Chest. 2008; 133(6Suppl):776S–814.
3. Rigau Comas D, Álvarez-Sabin J, Gil Núñez A, Abilleira Castells S, Borras Pérez FX, Armario García P, et al. Guía de práctica clínica sobre prevención primaria y secundaria del ictus. Med Clin (Barc). 2009;133:754–62.
4. Baigent C, Blackwell L, Collins R, Emberson J, Godwin J, Peto R, et al. Aspirin in the primary and secondary prevention of vascular disease: collaborative meta-analysis of individual participant data from randomised trials. Lancet. 2009;373:1849–60.
5. Reaume KT, Regal RE, Dorsch MP. Indications for dual antiplatelet therapy with aspirin and clopidogrel: evidence-based recommendations for use. Ann Pharmacother. 2008;42:550–7.
6. The European Stroke Organization (ESO) Executive Committee and the ESO Writing Committee. Guidelines for management of ischaemic stroke and transient ischaemic attack 2008. Cerebrovasc Dis. 2008;25:457–507.
7. Patrono C, Bachmann F, Baigent C, Bode C, De Catherina R, Charbonnier B, et al. Expert consensus document on the use of antiplatelet agents. Eur Heart J. 2004;23:166–81.
8. Llau JV, López-Forte C, Sapena L, Ferrandis R. Perioperative management of antiplatelet agents in non-cardiac surgery. Eur J Anaesthesiol. 2009;26:181–7.
9. Sierra P, Gómez-Luque A, Castillo J, Llau JV. Guía de práctica clinica sobre el manejo perioperatorio de antiagregantes en cirugía no cardiaca (Sociedad Española de Anestesiología y Reaniamción). Rev Esp Anestesiol Reanim. 2011;58(Supl 1):1–16.
10. Fleisher LA, Beckman JA, Brown KA, Calkins H, Chaikof E, Fleischmann KE, et al. ACC/AHA 2007 guidelines on perioperative cardiovascular evaluation and care for noncardiac surgery: executive summary. Anesth Analg. 2008;106:685–712.
11. Albaladejo P, Marret E, Piriou V, Samama CM. Perioperative management of antiplatelet agents in patients with coronary stents: recommendations of a French Task Force. Br J Anaesth. 2006;97:580–4.
12. Patrono C, Baigent C, Hirsh J, Roth G. Antiplatelet drugs. Chest. 2008;133:199S–233.
13. Collet JP, Montalescot G, Blanchet B, Tanguy ML, Golmard JL, Choussat R, et al. Impact of prior use or recent withdrawal of oral antiplatelet agents on acute coronary syndromes. Circulation. 2004;110:2361–7.
14. Burger W, Chemnitius JM, Kneissl GD, Rücker G. Low dose aspirin for secondary cardiovascular prevention –cardiovascular risks after its perioperative withdrawal versus bleeding risks with its continuation- review and meta- analysis. J Intern Med. 2005;257:399–414.
15. Biondi-Zoccai GG, Lotrionte M, Agostoni P, Abbate A, Fusaro M, Burzotta F, et al. A systematic review and meta-analysis on the hazards on discontinuing or not adhering to aspirin among 50,279 patients at risk for coronary artery disease. Eur Heart J. 2006;27:2667–74.
16. Chassot PG, Delabays A, Spanh DR. Perioperative antiplatelet therapy: the case for continuing therapy in patients at risk of myocardial infarction. Br J Anaesth. 2007;99:316–28.
17. Kearon C, Hirsh J. Management of anticoagulation before and after elective surgery. N Engl J Med. 1997;336:1506–11.
18. Doukekis JD, Berger PB, Dunn AS, Jaffer AK, Spyropoulos AC, Becker RC, et al. The perioperative management of antithrombotic therapy. Chest. 2008;133:299–339.
19. Grobler C, Callum J, McCluskey SA. Reversal of vitamin k antagonists prior to urgent surgery. Can J Anaesth. 2010. doi:10.1007/s12630-009-9250-3.

20. Douketis JD, Spyropoulos AC, Spencer FA, Mayr M, Jaffer AK, Eckman MH, Dunn AS, Kunz R. Perioperative management of antithrombotic therapy: antithrombotic therapy and prevention of thrombosis, 9th ed: American College of Chest Physicians evidence-based clinical practice guidelines. Chest. 2012;141:e326S–50.
21. Spyropoulos AC. Bridging of oral anticoagulation therapy for invasive procedures. Curr Hematol Rep. 2005;4:405–13.
22. Dunn A. Perioperative management of oral anticoagulation: when and how to bridge. J Thromb Thrombolysis. 2006;21:85–9.
23. Connolly SJ, Eikelboom J, Joyner C, Diener HC, Hart R, Golitsyn S, for the AVERROES Steering Committee and Investigators, et al. Apixaban in patients with atrial fibrillation. N Engl J Med. 2011;364:806–17.
24. Lopes RD, Alexander JH, Al-Khatib SM, Ansell J, Diaz R, Easton JD. Apixaban for reduction in stroke and other thromboembolic events in atrial fibrillation (ARISTOTLE) trial: design and rationale. Am Heart J. 2010;159(3):331–9.
25. Schulman S, Kearon C, Kakkar AK, Mismetti P, Schellong S, Eriksson H. Dabigatran versus warfarin in the treatment of acute venous thromboembolism. N Engl J Med. 2009;361: 2342–52.
26. Connolly SJ, Esekowitz MD, Yusuf S, et al. Dabigatran versus warfarin in patients with atrial fibrillation. N Engl J Med. 2009;361:1139–51.
27. The Einstein Investigators. Oral rivaroxaban for symptomatic venous thromboembolism. N Eng J Med. 2010;363:2499–510.
28. Patel MR, Mahaffey KW, Garg J, Pan G, Singer DE, Hacke W, the ROCKET AF Steering Committee, for the ROCKET AF Investigators, et al. Rivaroxaban versus warfarin in nonvalvular atrial fibrillation. N Engl J Med. 2011;365:883–91.
29. Eereberg E, Kamplhuisen PW, Sijpkens MK, Meijers JC, Buller HR, Levi M. Reversal of rivaroxaban and dabigatran by prothrombin complex concentrate. Circulation. 2011;124: 1573–9.
30. Levi M, Eerenberg E, Kamphuisen PW. Bleeding risk and reversal strategies for old and new anticoagulants and antiplatelet agents. J Thromb Haemost. 2011;9:1705–12.
31. Sié P, Samama C-M, Godier A, Rosencher N, Steib A, Llau JV, van der Linden P, Pernod G, Lecompte T, Gouin-Thibault I, Albadalejo P, Working Group on Perioperative Haemostasis; French Study Group on Thrombosis and Haemostasis. Surgery and invasive procedures in patients on long-term treatment with direct oral anticoagulants: thrombin or factor-Xa inhibitors. Recommendations of the Working Group on perioperative haemostasis and the French Study Group on thrombosis and haemostasis. Arch Cardiovasc Dis. 2011;104:669–76.
32. Llau JV, Ferrandis R, Castillo J, De Andrés J, Gomar C, Gómez-Luque A, Hidalgo F, Torres LM, en representación de los participantes en el Foro de Consenso de la ESRA-España de fármacos que alteran la hemostasia. Manejo de los anticoagulantes orales de acción directa en el periodo perioperatorio y técnicas invasivas. Rev Esp Anestesiol Reanim. 2012. http://dx.doi.org/10.1016/j.redar.2012.01.007
33. Available in: www.ema.europa.eu/docs/es ES/document library/EPAR - Product Information/human/000944/ WC500057108.pdf [Accessed 30 Apr 2012).
34. van Ryn J, Stangier J, Haertter S, Liesenfeld K-H, Wienen W, Feuring M, Clemens A. Dabigatran etexilate – a novel, reversible, oral direct thrombin inhibitor: interpretation of coagulation assays an reversal of anticoagulant activity. Thromb Haemost. 2010;103:1116–27.

Index

J.V. Llau (ed.), *Thromboembolism in Orthopedic Surgery*,   167
DOI 10.1007/978-1-4471-4336-9, © Springer-Verlag London 2013

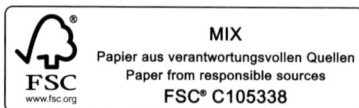

Printed by Books on Demand, Germany